The Complexity of Charaka's Ayurveda:

Looking at Charaka's System beyond New-Age Eyes

Durgadas (Rodney) Lingham, Veda Kovid

Published by:

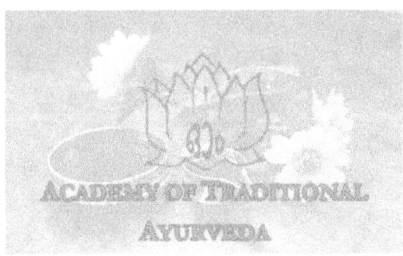

ACADEMY OF TRADITIONAL AYURVEDA

Title: The Complexity of Charaka's Ayurveda: *Looking at Charaka's System beyond New-Age Eyes*

ISBN-13: 978-1535176767
ISBN-10: 1535176768

Publisher: Academy of Traditional Ayurveda

Copyright Year: © 2017

Language: English

Country: New Zealand

DISCLAIMER:

The information and techniques provided in this book are not intended to diagnose, prescribe, treat or supplement as a cure or treatment for any medical condition and is purely for educational purposes alone and should never be considered as a supplement for medical conditions or diseases of any nature or kind.

One should always seek the advice of a qualified and Licensed Medical Professional for all health and medical conditions.

Table of Contents:

Foreword by Craig Williams (Indra Das)   i

Introduction   Page 1

I. A Brief History of Ayurveda   Page 3

I. The Background of Spiritual Ayurveda   Page 7

II. Rational Therapies and Genetics in Traditional Ayurveda   Page 11

III. Meditational and Yoga-related Disorders in Ayurveda   Page 15

IV. Understanding The Meaning of Prakriti   Page 29

IV. Ayurvedic Types Beyond the Three Doshic Types   Page 32

V. Antiquity of Ayurveda and Surgery in the Vedas   Page 40

VI. The Issue of Satmya (Suitability) in Ayurveda   Page 46

VII. Ayurveda and Insanity: A Fresh Look at the Classics from a Traditional Viewpoint   Page 48

VIII. Conclusion   Page 65

Further Discussions on Ayurveda's Science and New-Age Misconceptions: Page 71

I. Ayurvedic Microbiology: *An Historical Examination*   Page 72

II. Baseless Claims of Reiki and Pranic Healing   Page 81

III. Dispelling Marma Misconceptions: The Fallacy of *Siddha*   Page 87

IV. Meats and Their Use in Ayurveda   Page 96

Glossary   **Page 102**

Bibliography   **Page 107**

Foreword by Craig Williams (Indra Das):

The trajectory of the evolution of the medical system of *Ayurveda* in the West has been a precipitous journey. Initially viewed as an academic curiosity finding expression and attention in the milieu of academia and medical anthropology, *Ayurveda* has now emerged as a full-fledged burgeoning medical practice in the West. I remember first studying and learning *Ayurveda* during the early days of its cross-pollination into western soil. I was also deep into my journey of learning of Traditional Chinese Medicine and was inspired by the seemingly infinite potential of Eastern Medicine to offer a unique paradigm for global health. My academic background prior to my studies in *Ayurveda* were a combination of Philosophy, Religious Studies (with a focus on Hinduism) and Pre-med sciences. Due to this rather unconventional background, I was offered unique avenues of *Gurukula* education to complement what would be considered "classroom" studies instilling a great appreciation for the classical roots of *Ayurveda* and the deeper Traditional views of *Vaidika* systems.

Twenty-two years later, I would never have imagined the dismal state of contemporary *Ayurveda*. What was once a refined system of surgery and insightful clinical acumen has now become a New Age shibboleth. It's not uncommon to see the medical system of *Ayurveda* grouped together with such nebulous actions as: Reiki, Vibrational Healing, crystal therapy, tapping therapy and on and on. We can consider the traditional roots of *Ayurveda* related to the solar deity *Surya*. The further we move away from the Traditional roots of the original source texts of *Charaka, Sushruta and Vagbhata*, the farther we move away from the guiding authentic light of source teachings into the shadows of modern opinion and New Age obfuscation. When one examines these ancient source teachings, the modern New Age concepts are not hidden and waiting to be discovered; they are absent. Much like modern New Age archeology searches for the clues of "ancient aliens", the modern reader tends to superimpose shallow concepts and ideas onto ancient texts due to the lack of understanding of Sanskrit and the complex contextual integral systems of *Ayurveda, Yoga, Vedanta, Samkhya, Nyaya, Vaisheshika,* and *Mimamsa* to name just a few.

Why is this occurring? The issue is complex and there is not an easy cure. Much of the blame must be focused upon the teaching programs currently functioning as the gatekeepers of *Ayurvedic* education. In the majority of these programs scant attention is given to traditional texts outside of the occasional use of quotes and short excerpts. The students are not required to memorize and analyze the traditional texts and as a result end up with a watered-down representation of *Ayurveda* often supported by a combination of poor quality allopathic facts and a large serving of Quantum Physics added to avoid the dangers of critical thinking. Such students can speak of "chakras", "pranic healing" and hand out homogenized "dosha quizzes" yet are unable to intelligently discuss the history and nuances of Classical *Ayurveda* and apply this knowledge in a clinical setting.

However much of the blame must also be placed upon the teachers who are being held up as representatives of *Ayurveda* in the West. Why are these individuals not requiring students to learn the classics in-depth? Why are these teachers being promoted with Quasi-Guru status instead of the focus being upon the voluminous traditional teachings? In my opinion, these are the questions we must begin to ask if we expect the evolution of *Ayurveda* to sway from its current course of shallowing. For this shallowing to slow, we must begin to produce modern writings which are rooted in the teachings of Classical *Ayurveda* yet express a modern creativity which represents the eternal nature of *Ayurveda* without resorting to shallow New Age concepts or naïve connections to Quantum Physics. "*The Complexity of Charaka's Traditional Ayurveda*" is such a rare text. This text penetrates deep into the ancient history of *Ayurveda* and outlines a seemingly forgotten system of astounding complexity and clinical efficacy which bears no resemblance to the pasteurized and homogenized New Age *Ayurveda* marketed in spas and yoga studios.

The vast body of work produced by Durgadas Lingham is perhaps one of the most important modern reflections of the *Vaidika* light of *Surya,* radiating the ancient teachings in a modern vernacular free from the obfuscation of shallow New Age thought. His new text focuses on the important classical work *Charaka Samhita* and allows the reader to grasp ancient concepts which are far from antiquated or outdated. Writings such as this one shine a glimmer of hope in the dark age of the *Kali Yuga* and reminds us of the potential for a new dawn for *Ayurveda* in the western world. The work of Durgadas Lingham awakens the *Vaidika* Goddess of dawn, *Usha,* and ushers in hope for the future of *Ayurveda* beyond a stale allopathic rendering or a child-like New Age presentation. I hope all practitioners and most importantly teachers of *Ayurveda* read this important work and grasp its teachings.

Jai Agni!

-Craig Williams (Indra-Das)

Author: Tantric Physics Vol. 1: Cave of the Numinous and *Entering the Desert*

YogAyurvedAcharya

www.AyurvedaAustin.com

Introduction:

In the opening here, I would like to state that this project serves four purposes:

i. To show the ancient and advanced methods of Ayurveda and their origin in the most ancient of texts

ii. To reveal the integral nature of *Yoga, Jyotisha, Vastu* etc. as parts of the traditional and classical Ayurveda to enlighten people towards an Integral (*Purna*) Ayurveda system

iii. To deal with systems beyond the *three dosha* model commonly accepted in Ayurveda today, by revealing older schools of thoughts about *doshas* and *Prakriti* types and analysis

iv. To reveal how the New Age systems of Ayurveda often abuse the system through misunderstanding. In India, there are variations of Sanskrit pronunciation, but the western mispronunciations and butchering of these is not the same. The same goes with ill-founded, distorted and interpolated New Age concepts into Ayurveda today that also limit its scientific scope and teachings historically.

Traditional thinkers in India such as *Maharishi Dayananda Saraswati* and *Sri Aurobindo* held the ancient texts of the Vedas, including Ayurveda in high esteem. In more recent times also, my teacher, *Vedacharya Vamadeva Shastri* has also revealed the depth of Vedic and Ayurvedic wisdom, and his words, teachings and examples are also an inspiration, if not source, of this paper which deals and treats these subjects in a traditional manner allowing the reader to also cross-reference with textual references of tradition.

I hope in doing so, scholars East and West, naturopathic and allopathic will appreciate the greater depth and scope of which Ayurveda has to offer in the present day, as also the deeper integrated system explained, as per even the esoteric aspects of Ayurveda and their rational purpose in Ayurveda beyond some "magical mystery", to understand the deeper psyche behind such methods in Ayurveda as interconnected with the *darshanas* of *Yoga* and *Vedanta*, as also *Samkhya* on which it rests, as also these along with exoteric measures as counselling, herbal therapies, alchemical compounds and surgery, not simply, as in modern medicine, taking the latter and reducing it down to a system by itself, treating only half of the disease and not its cause.

- **Durgadas (Rodney) Lingham, Veda Kovid, R.A.P**
  Christchurch, NZ

Notes to the reader on translations used:

the *Vivekachudamani* of *Sri Shankaracharya* with translation by *Swami Madhavananda* has been sometimes employed and referenced also has been the *Hatha Yoga Pradipika* with translation by *Swami Muktibodhananda*. Referenced also and quoted are translations of *Sushruta Samhita, Sharngadhara Samhita, Ashtanga Hridayam* are of *K.R Srikanthamurthy; Charaka Samhita* of *P.V. Sharma*.

Kularnava Tantra of Ram Kumar Rai has also been referenced and translation employed where applicable.

A Brief History of Ayurveda:

Our history of Ayurveda starts with the Vedic civilization and the *Rig-Veda*, which mentions the ancient Physician-Gods, the *Ashwins* who restore people's eyesight, replace teeth, artificial limbs and rejuvenate people with the Soma, the *rasayana* anti-aging formulas. The text *Atharva Veda* (which has many hymns from the Rig-Veda) has specific hymns or *suktas* for various diseases and to herbs, noting their herbal properties and qualities, as well as microorganisms (*bhuta, asura, krimi*).

The three biological humours (*doshas*) in *Ayurveda* are called *tridhatu* in Ayurveda - "*dhatu*" meaning a constituent or stable substance and later meaning a tissue, metal etc. in *Ayurveda. Dosha* itself is referred to in the *Rigveda* first as a blemish, stain or disease, which is what it is connected to in the later *Charaka Samhita*. The three biological humours are *vata* (space and oxygen), *pitta* (fire and water) and *kapha* (water and earth), being wind, bile and phlegm respectively. These connect to the three cosmic forces in the *Vedas* as *Indra, Agni* and *Soma*, the deities of lightening and wind (*vayu*), fire and heat (*tejas*) and bliss, health and vitality (*ojas*) respectively.

In *Mehrgarh* around 7500BCE, Hindus were drilling teeth with bow-drills, being the first form of dentistry in the world.

Acharyas such as *Charaka* and *Sushruta* later arose with their own respective traditions. *Charaka's* school descended from the older school of *Purnavasu Atreya* and *Charaka's* work, *Charaka Samhita* was a redacted version of his Guru's work, the *Agnivesha Tantra*. *Sushruta's* work drew from the older teachings of *Divodasa Dhanvantari*. At their time, numerous other *Acharyas* also existed such as *Kashyapa, Bhela* etc. *Kashyapa's* work is known for Ayurvedic pediatrics. Other works as those of *Shalihotra* dealt with *Pashavayurveda* or Ayurvedic Veterinary science, especially relative to horses and elephants.

Here, *Ayurveda* became split into three main forms: *Manavayurveda* (Ayurveda for Humans), *Vrikshayurveda* (Botany Science) and *Pashvayurveda* (Veterinary Science), the roots of which are also in the *Vedas*. It also formed into eight branches (again, the roots of which can be found as early as the *Rig Veda*):

1. Kaya Chikitsa or Bodily Therapy, which aims at internal methods of healing the body
2. Shalya Tantra or Surgery
3. Shalyatantra or ENT Disorders
4. Kaumarabhritya or Pediatrics
5. Agadtantra or Science of Toxins
6. Bhutavidya or Science of Elements, relating to Psychology
7. Rasayana or Rejuvenation Therapy
8. Vajikarana or the Aphrodisiacs

While the *Sushruta* school laid more emphasis on *Shalyatantra* or surgery, the *Charaka* school laid more emphasis on *Kaya Chikitsa* or dealing with healing the body internally by correcting one's metabolism and various other regimes, such as *rasayana*. Both schools however employed all branches where required, including alchemy (*rasa-shastra*), which is related to the branches of *Agadtantra* and *Rasayana*.

Ayurveda was also the first to note of hospitals. *Charaka* notes that Ayurvedic hospitals must be set out with patients having their own rooms, attached bathrooms and pleasant music playing. The kitchen, pharmacy etc. are described in detail - right down to patient bedding and a water pot by his bedside! The world's oldest surviving hospital is in Sri Lanka at Mihintale and dates back to King Sena II around the 8th Century AD, however, records of earlier kings going back to 500BCE note of hospitals on Sri Lanka.

Sushruta's school was one of surgery that included many advanced methods as plastic surgery and describes some 300 surgical procedures, as well as the use of 120 types of surgical instruments and 1120 illnesses and their treatment. *Sushruta* also describes the unique method of using large ants as precursors to "surgical clips", that, being organic matter would disintegrate. The Buddha's physician, *Jivaka* around 600BCE is also known to have performed successful operations such as twisted bowels and also brain surgery.

Such novel techniques have become a great contribution to the world today. *Charaka* and *Sushruta* also describe Type1 and Type 2 diabetes for the first time. They are said to have lived around 2000 - 1500BCE.

Many modern methods as plastic surgery (Rhinoplasty) itself comes from Ayurveda, learnt by the British surgeon Joseph Constantine Carpue, who learnt this technique from the Ayurvedic surgeons of India based on ancient methods – aimed at reconstructing ears, noses and lips that were cut off in battle or fights in India. The current practice of rhinoplasty or plastic surgery of the nose is still known as the "Indian method", coined after *Sushruta*, who is also known as the "Father of Surgery" across the globe. *Sushruta* was not only a pioneer in these areas, but also taught students to practice first on vegetables to perfect their skills relative to careful incisions and also dissect human corpses to learn about anatomy.

Other complex operations for removing cancerous growths (*arbuda*) followed up with cauterization (today's modern method is Radiation therapy) , C-Sections, removal of Urinary stones, cataracts, removal of the prostate gland, repairing perforated intestines, drainage of fluids and more were performed in *Sushruta's* time about 4000 years ago as also a more complex form of Ayurvedic dentistry. His system came through from *Divodasa Dhanvanatri*, the incarnation of *Sri Dhanvantari Dev*, the patron deity of Ayurveda, said to have been born during the churning of the sea of milk in the Hindu *Puranas*.

Later from Sindh, around 500AD, came the great physician Vagbhata. His system is known in south India today as the *Ashtavaidya* system which fused local systems with his system in his *Ashtanga Hridaya* and *Ashtanga Sangraha*, that became the basis of Ayurveda in later India. His works drew from both *Charaka* and *Sushruta*, and his system included the surgical techniques and systems of *Sushruta*.

Later authors such as *Madhava* (700AD) with his *Madhava Nidana* work on diagnosis, *Sarngadhara* (14th Century) with his work on Ayurvedic herbal and mineral preparations and *Bhava Mishra* (1600AD) in his *Bhava Prakasha* - an updated work on the older classics that included new diseases as "foreign disease" (*pharingi-roga* or syphilis) are also noted.

Numerous commentaries on these main classics existed, as well as several other works. These however are considered the major texts, classified as the *brihat trayi* (greater traid) comprising *Charaka Samhita, Sushruta Samhita* and *Ashtanga Hridaya* and the *laghu trayi* or lesser triad, comprising the *Madhava Nidana, Sarngadhara Samhita* and *Bhava Prakasha*.

The earlier (greater) works were translated into Arabic around the 8th Century (Sushruta Samhita, known as *Kitab i Susrud* in Arabic) and Persian and Arabic in the 9th Century (Charaka Samhita, *Sharak* in Arabic). Ashtanga Hridaya was also translated into Arabic (*Asankar*). It was from the Arab world that these texts and their surgical techniques reached Europe. Around the 8th Century, many Indian Physicians such as *Manikya, Dhana* and *Bhela* came to Baghdad and taught and practiced at the Barmecides Hospital (named after the *Pramukh*, Arabic *Barmak* Buddhist family from the Balkh), following the Arab occupation in Sindh and transmission of information from east to west under the Abbasid Caliphate in Baghdad - these also included not only Hindu physicians, but also mathematicians, astronomer-astrologers, physicists and others. The non-Roman numerals and decimal place system, along with zero and many mathematical equations we use today came from Hindus living as teachers in Baghdad at the time. The Arabs were also familiar with the work of *Madhava* as well.

To show the skill and advanced nature of *Ayurveda*, the text "*Bhoja-prabandha*" of about 980AD deals with the life of the great King *Raja Bhoja*. In it, it was stated he was suffering from a brain tumour and two Ayurvedic surgeons were brought to him. Using a special drug, they made him unconscious, opened his skull, took out the tumour and then restored the skull with special Ayurvedic techniques and with another medicine, brought him back to consciousness. After this, *Raja Bhoja* was fine and lead a normal life, free from any complications. Hence, not only was brain surgery well-known in Ayurveda, but also medicines that induced comas and reversed the effects for complex operations also.

During the Muslim period in India from the 12th Century onwards, due to a lack of patronage, *Ayurveda* declined in India and became a system more or less limited to village *vaidyas* or physicians. Some areas however did continue these - as noted with the 16th Century work of *Bhava Mishra* and others such as *Madanpala* and those such as *Sayanacharya*, the great commentator on the *Vedas* during the *Vijayanagara Empire* in southern India that patronized Vedic sciences. While it also suffered during the British Raj, the subtle influence of surgeons as through Joseph Constantine Carpue took place and then a revival again afterwards with the formation of the BAMS (Bachelor of Ayurvedic Medicine and Surgery) in India and the many Indian Gurus that started bringing teachings to the west of the ancient medical system of Ayurveda, through which it has become of interest to many people lay in the west and physicians alike.

$\cdots$
6

I.The Background of Spiritual Ayurveda:

The view of the ancient system of *Charaka* and his system of Ayurveda from
the *Atreya* lineage going back to *Rishi Atreya* and his sons, *Soma Rishi* (also Moon), great
Yogi, *Dattatreya* and *Durvasa Rishi,* is considered one of herbal therapies, magical
therapies and treatments, when in fact, it is a highly sophisticated system; the doctrine
of his karma behind diseases does not ignore, but is interwoven into the genetic factors
he mentions behind disease. It should also note noted that, for the first time in
history, *Charaka* identifies Type 1 and Type 2 diabetes.

While the modern treatment of Ayurveda tends to favour the inner medicine of Charaka
(viz. *Daivavyapashraya, Yuktivyapashraya* and *Sattvavajaya - Charaka. Sutra.* XI. 54). Of
these, *daiva-vyapashraya* means use of
mantras, *oshadhi* (herbs), *mani* (gemstones), *mangala* (auspicious
acts), *bali* (offerings), *upahara* (gifts), *homa* (fire sacrifices), *niyama* (observances of
Yoga), *prayaschitta* (atonement), *upavasa* (fasting), *swastyayana* (auspicious rites), *pran
ipatagamana* (repeatedly going and offering obeisances, as in planets, Gurus, deities
etc.) etc.; *yukti-vyapashraya* means *ahara* or intake of foods and *aushadha-
dravyas* (herbal drugs or medicines) and *sattvavajaya* described as "*manonigraha*"
(controlling the mind).

From this, we can also deduct that mantra-therapies, potentialisation of herbs along
with Vedic rituals, *poojas* and offerings to the deities as in later Tantra and older
Vedic *yajnas, niyamas* of Yoga, use of gemstones, hence implying *Jyotisha* or astrological
and exotic measures as per chart energies of the planets, transits and *dasha* (planetary
periods and cycles) is also indicated here under spiritual therapies and the *Vaidya* or
physician was also required to know these also. This does not mean simply using
gemstones for healing as per their psycho-physical effects, but suitability of specific
gemstones as per planetary weaknesses and strengths to pacify them in one's birth-
charts in astrology to avoid subtle afflictions represented by these planets
(*grahas,* "seizers", meaning they prevent one from moving on karmically unless
pacified) and them first being *shuddhi* (purified) and infused with *shakti* or
potentialised first. This is an example of how the New-Age implementation of these
gemstones fails to match that of the more complex traditional approach. It also follows
no other auxiliary rituals mentioned here by Charaka also, as reverence (of planets,
planetary deities etc.) and other methods.

As an example, the effects of gemstones, as they help in afflicting and weak planets,
representing our karmic potentials in the charts in the science of *Jyotisha* or astrology,
help strengthen weaker ones and pacify those afflicting or too strong, when properly
energised, purified and worn touching the skin of the body, therefore acting in a
more *saukshmika* (subtle), not physical manner in treating disease, i.e. the *mulakarma-
nidanas* or the root-karmic causes behind disease (whether congenital or due
to *doshas* etc.) - one karma has been reduced, so also diseases can be cured. This is why
gemstones have such effects in healing, but not when used topically or physically alone,
for their power, so says even the classics, is their *prabhava* or special (subtle) action,
which is *achintya* (inconceivable to the mind) - *Charaka, Sutra,* XXVI.70. Herbs also have
this as also other remedies - as an example given, *visha* (poison) is also a *vishaghna-*

mukta (anti-poisonous and immunity / freedom) for poison also (*Charaka, Sutra,* XXVI.69). Relating to planets then, those with afflicted Mercury and Moon, wearing stones for these planets (emerald and pearl respectively) would hence help in psychological and nervous / neurological disorders, such as Parkinsonism, but not physically, but due to strengthening afflicted / weaker planets on a subtle level. This is how the *mani-prabhava* or special power of gemstones is to be understood. While rejected by some groups in Hinduism as the *Arya Samaj,* they also acknowledge that karma exists and employ methods as *pranayama* and *homa* to impart *sattvas* or purity and reduce karma, which is, in no way at all, different to what we describe here relative to gemstones.

Continuing from the aforementioned mentioned therapies, *Upahara* also includes gifts of clothes, gold, cattle, sacred images etc. to Brahmins and others one had offended in past lives to atone for karma (behind genetic diseases, as we shall discuss later on), as also *upavasa* etc. as part of *prayaschitta.* Such methods also include prayers to Varuna in the Rig Veda and also aspects as offerings of cattle, gold etc. in the Rig Veda, which are also perhaps indicative of these practices in ancient Vedic times as part of healing in disease also. *Bali* and *Homas* are also special Tantric and Vedic rites that appease various deities, ancestors, planets etc. to help reduce one's karmic "debts" and to be used along with the previously discussed therapies as well. (It should be noted here, the concepts of integers or negative numbers originated in ancient India by the mathematician *Brahmagupta* who represented them as debts). *Niyamas* are the positive observances in Yoga disciple that *Charaka* also mentions as part of these treatments, viz. *Shaucha* - purity (in mind, body and speech), *Santosha* - contentment, *Tapas* - austerities (as fasts, sacred festivals, pilgrimages etc.), *Swadhyaya* - self-study (meaning study of sacred texts to impart purity to the mind etc. from *Vedas, Puranas, Agamas / Tantras, Yoga / Vedantic* texts and their commentaries etc.) and *Ishvarapranidhana* or devotion to the deity (under which *poojas, homas, bali, yajnas, japa, mantra* etc. occur) on a daily basis. The primary aspects of Yoga hence play a part in Ayurveda (*yamas* and *niyamas* take years, if not decades of mastery before the body can be stilled through *Asana* or seated posture (hence why *Ishvarapranidhana,* devotion to the deity is important first, for their grace as also purification of the mind first to have such stability).

This explains the complexity of *daiva chikitsa / vyapashraya,* beyond mere placing of gemstones on the body and a few generic mantras!

We must also make a note here relative to the modern "chakra-balancing" and "energy healing" movements. These generally follow no guidelines of working with the deities, no strict diets to purify one's inner *prana* (life-force) or *shakti* (celestial power as the Divine Mother) from which such healing power derives, after several decades of practice of the above mentioned *sattvika* or *daivika* modalities by Charaka. It takes some Yogis several lifetimes, including decades of practice of awakening past-life impressions (*samskaras*) and therapies in the present life or incarnation. On this note, with relation to the *ashta siddhi* (eight mystical powers of Yoga), *Charaka* (*Sharira,* I. 140-41) states states these are only possible by *shuddha-sattva-samadhana* or concentration on the purified (*shuddha*) mind (*sattva*). Likewise, only when *rajas* and *tamas* are completely negated as also past-life karmas are also destroyed (*karma-samkshaya*) - esp. by aforementioned methods under *daiva chikitsa*, is *moksha* or liberation possible (Charaka, Sharira, I.142).

This is also echoed in the statements of *Acharya Sushruta* also, on reincarnation and *purvajanma-sanskara smarana* or remembrance of past-life traits:

"Those who had engaged in the study of shastras (sacred texts) in their previous birth becomes endowed with sattvas (quality of purity and clarity) and able to remember their previous lives. Karmas (actions) which a person performed in his earlier life, he will attain the same nature (guna) when he is born again" - **Sushruta Samhita, Sharira Sthana. II. 57-58**

It is hence clear from the Ayurvedic classics dealing with Yoga and healing, then, that one doesn't just simply decide in their fourties or fifties that they are born with healing powers; these traits will, if they are within the person and developed from past lives, display themselves at an early age. Cases are such as *Sri Ramana Maharishi*, who at the tender age of only sixteen, attained *Atmajnana* or Self-realisation, due to his past-actions. It also comes organically, naturally and inwardly, not simply learnt physically (although this can aid afterwards, or even stimulate one's past mental impressions beforehand). The point is, from a young age, one will be drawn to such spiritual practices deeply and have such experiences.

The texts also warn relative to nations as well, due to *adharma* (unrighteousness) and *prajnaparadha* (mistake of the intellect) due to past-life karmas etc. as also actions of those ruling and administering the nations, that plagues etc. can manifest as a result of these, as also bacteria and *rakshasas* or demonic entities (*Charaka, Vimana,* III.20, 22) as also diseases due to *shapa* (curses), which all stems from *adharma* or unrighteous behavior of individuals (further verse, 23; *Sushruta, Uttarasthana,* LX.5 further states on this that violating social rules, committing violence, uncleanliness etc. cause one to become afflicted by them). This is something we need to look at in the world today closely, since the behaviour of Europe and other nations historically and their karmas or collective *samskaras* (traits) formed by the rulers also ushered in many new diseases by ignoring righteousness and proper conduct, which also explains the new and *asadhya* (incurable) diseases we have today and epidemics globally. This is also why *desha* or land was examined in Ayurveda as per diseases, according to it's *dharma* or righteousness, climate, seasons and their effects on the *doshas*, as also the influences there regarding *gocharas* (planetary transits) on the land and also the individual etc. as a complex system of healing. This is also something that in ancient times, large-scale *yajnas* or *homas* - sacrifices and fire-ceremonies were performed to eliminate, both to (a) reduce karmic actions and *samskaras* subtly by atoning for them and (b) to help purify the air of airborne parasites and bacteria or viruses causing these.

Ayurveda is of the view that *krimija rogas* or virus-born diseases are also due to negative or *asuric* entities manifesting their negative presences, giving rise to their minute and airborne pathogens, hence both spiritual and physical therapies are required to completely uproot them, and their presence is also due to *karya-krana bhava*, the law of cause and effect, i.e. transgressions from one's past-lives causing such afflictions to manifest. These ideas are seen commonly in the *Atharva Veda*, but first mentioned relative to health and *doshas* in the *Rig Veda*, where the Sun-God, *Surya* (also King of the plants) is invoked, with his heat and light to dispel them:

"The Deva expels all the rakshasas and yatudhanas, with all those offensive defects (prati-dosham, Vikriti) and hatred." **Rig Veda. I.35.10**

Rakshasas are those who injure, destroy etc. *Yatudhanas* are another class of *rakshasas*. *Prati-dosham* can also mean the "offensive *dosha*", or the vitiated *dosha* (*vikara*), depending on how we translate the term. In the context of viruses and bacteria, the Ayurvedic classics, such as *Sushruta Samhita* also have charms and special fumigation rituals to help protect against them, especially post-surgery, where they are seen to attack a person whose wounds are exposed or ulcerating, thus perhaps also the cause behind cancers manifesting today from cysts removed and surgeries - the term used again is *rakshasa*, By contrast, ancient methods after operative procedures (*Charaka, Chikitsa*, XXV, 101-106) included *agnikarma* (thermal cauterisation) or *kshara* (alkali cauterisation) of the area, followed by pouring hot ghee or bee's wax on the area and suturing, which prevented air or bacteria getting into the wound, as well as placing the patient in a specially fumigated room or chamber, where hymns were chanted etc. to prevent or ward off negative entities causing physical airborne bacteria. Ancient post-operative procedures were hence much more advanced and hygienic than today's methods!

Abhisanga-jwara or fever for example, caused by lust (*kama*), grief (*shoka*), fear (*bhaya*) or anger (*krodha*) or *abhishakta* (negative microorganisms) in *Charaka* (*Chikitsa*, III.114-117) is also related to poisonous air and *bhutas* (negative astral entities). Here, the mental factors are causative, the *bhutas* or negative entities are related to the microorganisms or negative entities they cause, which hence vitiate the air or environment, causing such fevers and diseases. The primal cause again however are past-life factors and deeds (*Charaka, Chikitsa*, III.13-14).

The Ayurvedic model then, is explained as follows:
Amaja Ahara (intake of toxic foods) > *Manovahasrota malas* (wastes in the mental channels causing darkness and dullness of perception or *viveka- discrimination)*
> *Prajnaparadha* (mistake of the intellect)
> *Adharma* (committing unrighteous behavior and actions) > *Karmaja* (karmic effects, which also include *Sahaja* or congenital factors in future births), which in turn attracts the *Rakshasas* (negative life-force or harmful astral entities) > *Tamasic Prana* (negative life-force and air polluted by *rakshasas*) > *Krimija* (airborne parasites and bacteria or viruses form as a result of *tamasic prana*) > *Roga* (disease).

Science sadly stops only at the *bheda* or manifestation stage and does not consider the *mula-nidanas* or primal causative factors behind these in the ethers, which have *karmic* effects from past and also present lives, but the cause of even these *karmic* factors is due to diet etc., causing the mind to act incorrectly, due to vitiation of the intellect (*prajna*). Thus, Ayurveda gives a proper scope for these, providing the full picture, not simply the end-result and physical manifestation alone without answers which modern science and medicine, like Abharamic faiths they tried to reject, but were tainted by, fail to address by remaining silent on them also.

II. Rational Therapies and Genetics in Traditional Ayurveda:

While these exotic measures and deeper subjects are treated by Charaka, he also mentions, for vitiated doshas in the body (*sharira-dosha-prakopa*, Ch. Sutra. XI. 55), three therapies which include *anta parimarjana* (internal cleansing), *bahi marjana* (external cleansing) and *shastra-pranidhana* (surgical operation). *Anta parimarjana* means diet and herbal therapies; *bahi marjana* means *abhyanga* (massage) etc. and *shastra-pranidhana* or surgical operation that of ten therapies mentioned by Charaka (Ch. Sutra, XI.55),
viz, *chedana* (excision), *bhedana* (piercing), *vyadhana* (puncturing), *darana* (rupturing), *lekhana* (scraping), *utpatana* (extraction), *pracchana* (scarification), *sivana* (suturing), *k shara* (alkalis) and *jalauka* (leeches). These are also mentioned elsewhere as *patana* (incision), *vyadhana* (puncturing), *chedana* (excision), *lekhana* (scraping), *prac hana* (scarification) and *sivana* (suturing). (*Chikitsasthana*, XXV.55) (56-60). *Charaka* also describes the *Sushruta* technique of repairing perforated intestines, by using ants as surgical clips before suturing them again (*Charaka, Chikitsasthana,* XIII.184.188).

We must note these sections were revised by *Dridhabala* in the 4th Century AD but still draw from older sources (*Agnivesha Tantra* and *Charaka Samhita* of *Charaka*). *Dridhbala's* is the last "edited" work we have in existence and he "reconstructed" the latter missing parts of *Charaka Samhita*, drawing from older texts (*Charaka, Chikitsasthana,* XXX.289-291, *Siddhisthana*, XII.36-40, 52-54) and hence reconstructed the original teachings of 120 chapters of *Agnivesha Tantra* (*Siddhisthana,*XII.34).

Thus, six forms of treatment are mentioned by *Charaka*, the so-called propagator of "internal medicine" alone, who deems internal therapies (*anta parimarjana*), as but one of these six systems and also, spiritual therapies or *daiva vyapashraya* as also but one of the six also, going back to the original *Atreya sampradaya* of Ayurveda that *Charaka* worked on, himself redacting the older *Agnivesha Tantra* (that it appears, *Dridhbala* et al also worked from to reconstruct *Charaka*'s missing portions).

We know that the *Sushruta* school of surgeons perfected rhinoplasty, otoplasty, cataract surgery, perforated intestines and several others, from which the Western variations of these also derived historically [1]. The gift of surgery to the world from Ayurveda is hence often understated, seeing it as merely a system of the '*daiva-vyapashraya*' aspect alone, when in fact, as seen from *Charaka's* own testimony, it forms one of only six of his therapies, of which, he mentions ten surgical ones alone.

Charaka was also not simply about doshas. He also knew genetics well and stated that any actions the Mother does, such as foods eaten, behavior, vitiated doshas and past deeds of the individual - all can bring about doshic and organ abnormalities or diseases (*vikaras*) (*Charaka Samhita, Sharirasthana*, II.29-30). As such, any actions or influences such as violent of the mother, bad thoughts or actions, alcoholism etc., as we know, will affect the child and the doshas. Thus, many today, coming from violent homes with alcoholic issues will according to Ayurveda, be contributing factors for creating a disposition of vata disorders, if not *Prakriti* itself, as such factors aggravate vata!

Charaka also talks about the genetic factors behind diseases and the origin of them in *karmaja* (past-life actions) as a cause of these. When *asadhya* (incurable), methods as under *daiva-vyapashraya* are hence indicated to negate them, due to these genetic defects, caused by past-life actions (as there is no 'effect' *without* a 'cause' says Ayurveda; congenital disorders are not simply random fate, they also have a nidana or cause, so says *Charaka* et al).

Leucoderma (Sanskrit, *Switra, Kilasa*), a skin condition, for example, is a disease caused by insults to teachers, gods, impious activities, previous karmas and incompatible foods as per the ancient Ayurveda classics (*Charaka Samhita, Chikitsasthana,* VIII.177), as also other skin disorders (VIII.4-8). *Unmada* or insanity due to psychic possession is also caused by negative karmic actions (*Charaka Samhita, Nidanasthana,* VII.10, VII.19-20).

Twins and such, as also difficulties in pregnancy are due to previous karmas (*Charaka Samhita, Sharirasthana,* II.12-16), causing also differentiation in twins. In cases of hermaphrodites etc., Vata gets disturbed and causes disorders, also due to previous actions (further verses 18-21). The same is also due to children that are born with genetic defects also, due to *rajasic* and *tamasic samskaras* or agitating and dark tendencies which create or form the embryo accordingly (discussed in further verses 29-36).

One's birth constitution and formation as per genetics can hence be understood deeply from the following verses from Charaka, but as noted however, Ayurvedic classics that the cause of these effects or disorders, is karmic and due to negative karmic actions in the past (*Charaka Samhita, Nidanasthana, VII.10, VII.19-20*). Likewise, while Ayurveda recognises that *atmaja* (genetic) disorders derives from the ovum or sperm or mother or father, the primal or *karana* (causal) form of this is also karmic, and causes afflictions as a result in the embryo, as also to the psyche:

"All foetuses have four elements (all except ether – viz. wind, fire, water and earth) which are fourfold also as maternal, paternal, nutritional and self-borne. Because of them the dominant factors arise from past-life deeds of the parents and resemble the physical appearance. Likewise the mental state is also determined by the past lives or species."
-Charaka Samhita, Shaririasthana, II.23-27

"Deeds in previous lives are known as 'Daiva' (divine) and those from the present life as 'Paurusha' (pertaining to man). These in an unbalanced manner cause disease, when in balance they avoid them." **-Charaka Samhita, Sharirasthana, II.44**

"Past karmas are called 'Daiva' (karmas) and are observed as the cause of diseases in time. There is no great karma (action) in which the fruit is not enjoyed (reaped). Diseases caused by karmaja (karmic factors) neutralise therapeutic measures and subside only on the destruction of deeds (which have caused them)." **-Charaka Samhita, Sharirasthana, I.116-117**

Ayurveda thus considers the genetic factors caused by karma in diseases also, including Lesbianism. *Charaka* (*Chikitsasthana*, XXX.34) states that lesbianism is due to a genetic factor in which Vata afflicts the ovaries in the embryo, causing this condition. What is striking here is that there is a link, as modern science has shown a higher rate of Polycystic Ovaries among Lesbian as opposed to heterosexual women [2]. The common term used in the texts to describe genetic defects is bijadosha, which literally means "vitiation of the seed", sometimes translated as a disorder of the ovum.

The classics also mention other genetic diseases, including hereditary diabetes (*Charaka*, *Chikitsasthana*, VII.57, note terms *kulaja* - familial, *jatah* - genetic and *bijadosha* - affliction of the seed); piles (*Charaka*, *Chikitsasthana*, XIV.5-8) and even disorders relating to the semen and impotency (*Charaka*, *Chikitsasthana*, XXX.190).

The ancient science of Ayurveda has a deep understanding of genetic factors and also the doshas causing the afflictions to the sperm and ovum or embryo, thus creating abnormalities in the foetus, but all of this derived from past-life causative factors, not simply random fate or no explanation for this. Hence, as noted, spiritual therapies are here required to alter one's "subtle DNA" if we like, or their karmic impressions to modify the (genetic) outcome of the physical body, which otherwise, becomes incurable. Thus, such therapies should be considered in severe and congenital cases, those of juvenile diseases (diabetes, cancer etc.) as per the Ayurvedic model, along with the other exoteric treatments to be wholly effective. Here also, in the highest path of *Jnana-Yoga* is elaborated by *Charaka* (*Sharira*, V.7, esp. V. 13-26) by disassociating with the body by seeing the cosmos and all deities as but reflections of one's own Self and the cosmos as the Self-reflected, starting with seeing the divinities and concepts within the body itself (*Charaka*, *Sharira*, V.5).

III. Meditational and Yoga-related Disorders in Ayurveda:

We have discussed the *Ashta-siddhi* or eight mystical powers in Yoga before. However, it is time here to make a note that the *Ashta-siddhis* are also not simply gained by Yoga. They can also manifest as a result of psychic possession or meditational disorders, creating superhuman speech, valour, power and movements and also knowledge (*jnana*) and understanding (*vijnana*), are caused by *bhutonmada* (possession caused by spirits or astral entities), as a result of past-life actions (*Charaka, Chikitsasthana,* IX.15-16).

Relating to *bhaya* (fear), *shoka* (grief) etc. noted by *Charaka* as being causative factors under mental disorders here also relates to certain visions, caused by awakening the *Kundalini* or opening of lower chakras or even *patalachakras* (the lower chakras), which open us up to negative astral forces. These can also cause diseases and mental disorders:

i. Talatala Chakra: Talatala Loka, 'Realm of Non-being' and ruled by Venus or Asuramaya, representing materialism

This is the lower manifestation of the *Sahasrara-Padma* or Crown Chakra, located in the body in the top of the skull. It is the highest of these lower chakras.

It corresponds to the **Asura** or demon-type personality. Such people are very monumental and have much wealth, courage but also traits of anger, and jealously and can be gluttons. Such a temperament is a materialistic businessperson who is overweight and has wealth and power in society and seeks to keep it that way! *Asuras* can be very devotional to the Gods, which makes them a higher type under the lower levels of Consciousness.

ii. Sutala Chakra: Sutala Loka, Realm of Spiritual Darkness, ruled by *Bali Maharaj* and *Danavas*

This is the lower manifestation of the *Ajna* or Third-chakra, located in the body between the brows in Yoga. Whereas the *Ajna Chakra* is the chakra of spiritual knowledge, the *Sutala Chakra* reflects it as that of spiritual ignorance. *Sutala Chakra* or *Loka*, the sphere connects to the *Rakshasa* personality and is the personality of back-biting and egotism with a lust for meats.

A **Rakshasa** type is a more worldly *Sattvic-based* or higher type under the *rajasic* personalities below the *Asura.* Such a person is like an Asura type but of a lower kind and capable of understanding things by themselves but more terrifying and jealous in nature that often has a large ego and often transgresses the social norm or laws. Such people are the typical white-collar criminals and such of society who take pride in ripping off the system or the tax-man and feel no remorse in doing so!

iii. Vitala Chakra: Vitala Loka, Realm of Confusion and confused beings, often compared to the state of atheists or Buddhists.

This is the lower manifestation of the *Vishuddha* or Throat-chakra, located in the body in the middle of the throat. It represents here confusion over speech and translations and hence the realm of confusion, delusion and atheism. It reflects the higher element of Ether or Space which they confuse as being the void (*shunya*). The *Vitala Chakra* relates to the *Pishacha* type of personality.

The **Pishacha** type person scavenges foods which have been left behind are not shy and are very lustful. Such people we can see with criminals in society or the homeless who move from place to place and scrounges for food off the streets and by begging.

iv. Atala Chakra: *Atala Loka,* Realm of Fear, and having no end. Realm of the *Narakas* or Hells, where temporal punishment is administered.

This is the lower manifestation of the *Anahata* or Heart-chakra, located in the body in the chest area. It is not to be confused with the spiritual heart-*chakra* – *Hridaya Chakra*, which is located at the right of the body, representing the Sun and the Self. It reflects the higher element of Air.

This category or sphere, the *Atala Chakra* is the realm of the **Sarpa-type** of personality – that of a Serpentine-type personality.
Such people are fickle-minded, fast in nature, always changing place or abode, angry and aggressive, deceptive and like recreational pastimes. We see such people as people who have undergone severe mental trauma or drug abuse in life, but seek to blame others for their predicament. They seldom seek help and when they do, they are seldom successful due to the waves of previous *rajasic samskaras* (rajasic traits or tendencies) from the past mixed with the *rajasic samskaras* in this life that they have picked up and added to their state. They can be intelligent however!

v. Rasatala Chakra: *Rasatala Loka*, Realm of materialism and hence demonic heavenly realms, comparable to the worlds of the Gods.

This is the lower manifestation of the *Manipura* or Fire-chakra, located in the body in the solar-plexus. It reflects the higher world or element of Fire and *Manipura* itself means the 'City of Gems', which in the netherworlds is a heavenly paradise far more opulent than the *Swargas* or the heavens of the Gods.

The Rasatala Chakra represents the more **Preta type** of personality – that of a ghostly figure.

Such a type is lazy, possessive, jealous, and sensuous and likes to hoard things and not give anything to others. Such types are always plagued by anxiety and distress. Such types are those who hard that much that they turn their homes or environments into living garbage tips and never seek to remove their clutter. Their wealth becomes their downfall.

vi. Mahatala Chakra: *Mahatala Loka*, Great confusion realm or of Ego. Egoistic demonic species that feed off arrogance and pride.

This is the lower manifestation of the *Swadhisthana* Water-chakra, located in the lower abdominal region of the bladder or the *basti marma*, the pressure point as it is known in Ayurvedic medicine. It reflects the higher element of water, of which itself also relates to the mind (*manas*) – itself of a watery nature and prone to confusion.

The *Mahatala Chakra* realm is that of the **Shakuna** or bird-type personality and always fleeting or agitated.

Such a type is mobile like a bird and does not stay in one play long and always distressed and always impatient and always consuming foods. It is placed just above the purely *tamasic* types owing to it being a bird - an animal.

vii. *Patala Chakra*: *Patala Loka*, Realm of wickedness. Cruel beings dwell here, such as lesser classes of demons ('aliens') inimical to humans and other beings.

This is the lower manifestation of the *Muladhara* or Root and Earth-chakra, located in the body at the base of the spine.

Patala-Chakra is the realm of the **Pashava** or beastly-type personality in Ayurveda and Yoga.

Such people always think negative thoughts, are slow in whatever they do, has many dreams and is lustful as well as denying their own issues and problems. Such people are very difficult to be helped and are sloths and act like animals.

By entering these states, or chakras, through deep sleep, meditation etc. we can hence attain astral travel. Fear, sickness and near-death can also cause these, and hence the prime time demons in ancient beliefs, came to harass humans, the negative beings encountered in Yoga and hence one can confuse the functioning of the higher chakras with these lower ones, which, if the body is not first purified along with the mind, can cause difficulties, as stated by *Charaka*.

We can also see from these how most people, even in Yoga circles actually fall into these categories of the lower chakras, rather than the higher chakras of which they claim to be working with. These are some of the dangers of working with the chakras and mantras, especially without proper guidance, diets and lifestyles to complement them!

We must note that traditional authors caution on *Kundalini* and also the *chakras* and viewing them as physical [3].

Often in Yogic practices, these are due to the body not being purified first.
Under *shaucha*, *Hatha-Yoga* employs a range of techniques to purify the mind-body complex, but only if there is excess mucous or toxins in the body first. Yet, purity of the mind-body complex and hence *Sattvic prana* or pure life-force must first be attained before working with the *chakras* or any Yogic practices (as even *pranic healing*) at an inner level, or it becomes a mere mental exercise, or can, as noted, even open up one to

negative occult or astral realms which also provide at times mystic powers, but without proper *viveka* or discrimination, one is unable to discern where these are coming from; this also comes under the greater *bhuta-graha* or possession by lesser entities of Ayurveda.

Certain Yogic practices when forced can also bring on diseases.

As an example, in weaker *Vata* types, such practices may harm people:

"If there be excess of fat or mucous in the body, the six kinds of practise (kriyas) should be performed first. But others, not suffering from the excess of these, should not perform them. **(Hatha Yoga Pradipika, II. 21)**

It is hence clearly mentioned here that unless one is suffering from excess phlegm (*shleshma*) or fat (*medas*), as in the case of obesity, or diseases of a *Kapha* (phlegmatic nature) according to Ayurvedic medicine, they should not be performed.

The six practices are:

1. *Neti*, meaning cleansing the nose, which was done either through *Jala-neti* (a water-pot filled with saline solution in each nostril) and also *Sutra-neti*, in which this was done by inserting a thread into the nose to help in breathing and cleanse all toxins and build-up from the nasal cavities and sinuses.

Cautions: Cautions must be noted here when using saline solutions, especially for *vata* types, which can be excessively drying to the sinuses. In winter, a little ginger can be used to clear excess *kapha* and for *Vata*, medicated oils are better, even if to follow-up after *neti*, which include formulas such as *anu taila*, which can also be used for *pitta* and inflamed sinuses, as also medicated ghees.

2. *Dhauti* to cleanse the stomach, which involved the swallowing of cloths and also *Vamana* or vomiting procedures to eliminate the build-up of *kapha* of phlegm from the stomach-region, creating an upward-movement.

Cautions: This is a dangerous process and hence, to remove phlegm, *vamana* or medicated vomiting is better, with special decoctions of licorice milk etc. Otherwise this can aggravate conditions and be very dangerous as also, by excessively drying and depleting to *vata* and disturb the movement of *udanavayu* or the up-moving air.

3. *Basti* or enemas for cleansing the colon, in which tubes were inserted and one would suck water up into the colon and release it to stop *Vata* or wind getting accumulated along with *ama* or toxins in the colon.

Cautions: Medicated *bastis* are of two types: *anuvasana* or oleated and *Kashaya* or medicated formulas. The former is better where there is dryness and the latter where there are blockages in the stool etc. to loosen it. One should not overly use water alone and such solutions, as it can be too drying by itself to the colon, and mixtures of sesame or medicated oils are better to lubricate the colon and prevent drying.

4. *Trataka* or Yogic-gazing, by which tears would flow upon looking at a candle for some time and helped cleanse the eyes (*akshi-shodhana*) and also the liver and emotions also, helping to release various *vasanas* of mental impressions in the mind, especially those connected to lust (*kama*) and anger (*krodha*).

5. *Bhastrika* or breathing like bellow-movements, a form of *Pranayama* or breathing technique to throw toxins from the body and awaken the *pranagni* or the fire of breath so that one's breath in Yoga was then more *Sattvic* or pure in state and promoted a good state of mind and healing also. This technique helps cleanse the *nadis* or subtle channels in the Yoga system, as also does *Siddhasana*, as we discussed under *Asana*.

Cautions: *Bhastrika* can be too heating in summer and hotter climates, as also to *pitta* and also deranging to *vata* in excess and better for *kapha*. Alternative nostril breathing is better for *vata* here and left nostril breathing for *pitta* to cool them down, along with mantras *om* (on inhalation), *vam* (on retention) and *ram* on exhalation for *vata* and for *pitta*, *sham* and *shreem* on inhalation and exhalation, with *yam* on retention.

6. *Nauli* or abdominal movements to help the *jatharagni* or digestive fire, which in *Hatha-Yoga*, the forceful Yoga system that requires much exercise, caused high *Vata* (wind) in people and so these exercises were done daily to ensure that *Vata* did not accumulate, especially in non-*Pitta* individuals who had variable digestions and were aggravated by this Yoga.

Cautions: This can be difficult for *kapha* types and so stronger spices and formulas such as *trikatu* are better for them internally. This is better and easier for *vata* types and *pitta* types should moderate this, unless they are on heavy dairy and raw-food diets, such as in *Sattvic* Yogic diets, in which this help them awaken the digestive fire.

These constitute the cleansing of the body or the awakening of the *dehika-agni* or the fire of the body with regards to purity, but we must also awaken the *shauchika manasika-agni* also or the fire of mental purity as well which means to avoid thinking badly of or harshly others (*paurushyam*), jealousy and such also.

Trataka, that is, Yogic gazing, at a ghee lamp or deity image or picture until the eyes begin to water, helps with *nirodha* (calmness or controlled state) of the mind (especially excess *Pranavayu* or Vata / Wind in the head region causing anxiety, hyperactivity etc.) through developing one-pointedness (*eka-gra*). It also helps awaken the intellect (*buddhi*) by awakening discrimination (*viveka*), itself the key to proper mental health, by governing the "mental metabolism" so to speak. Just as unwanted food wastes in our GI tract causes discomfort and diseases, so also in the mind, *vasanas* or mental impressions likewise, if not burnt up or discriminated, cause issues.

Trataka is hence a very useful tool in healing the mind and is fine for use. It works well when one also does *Vasana daha tantra*, that is, writing down all one's mental worries and burning it. It's a kind of "mental emesis" (*manasika vamana* in Sanskrit).

Still, we must take the warning here and realise that such practises themselves, unless one is suffering from specific diseases, should be avoided, for the better health of the person, or Yogi!

These also include the practise of *Kapala Bhati*, which is a special abdominal-related Pranayama or breathing technique, by which the air is forcefully pushed from the body via the abdomen.

Likewise, the methods *Charaka* mentioned
under *niyamas* including *Ishvarapranidhana* etc. also relate to helping calm the mind-body complex before going into higher limbs as *Asana* (postures)
and *Pranayama* (breathing techniques) or the mind cannot be stilled.

Pranayama:

The *Yoga-Sutras* or *Patanjali* (II.50) describe *pranayama* as the three aspects of external and internal flow of the breath, with the third being stillness or cessation of the breath itself by which the cessation of *vrittis* (fluctuations of the mind) are stilled, regulated by time, and place, by which the breath is made to be slow or prolonged and subtle.

Hence, *pranayama* must be developed slowly and not forced. It cannot be done to forcibly hold the breath as in many modern methods, which can cause mental issues. The fourth *pranayama* however is beyond these states (II.51), where the flow of breath is continuous and karmic veils are negated (II.52; II.12). It is hence a prerequisite to attain this state after several years of practice (not force) before even attempting *dhyana* or meditation, before which *pratyahara* (withdrawal of senses, as also from impressions as food, toxic lifestyles etc. must be practiced) and *dharana* (concentration, making the mind single-pointed and focused) have to be attained.

Before *pranayama* however, *asana* or posture has to be developed, by stilling the body, hence the mind (*manas*) and hence therefore the senses (*indriyas*). Forcing any of these disturbs *vata* in the mind and body and causes injuries, psychological disturbances and others.

Hence, *Pranayama* can cause diseases and disorders when not performed properly or done forcefully:

"Just as lions, elephants and tigers are controlled by and by, so the breath is controlled by slow degrees, otherwise it kills the practiser himself. When breath-control (pranayama), etc., are performed properly, they eradicate all diseases; but an improper practice generates diseases.
(Hatha Yoga Pradipika, II. 15-16)

The *Tantric* texts also note the importance of these **(Kularnava Tantra):**

"A Yogic breathing technique (pranayama) devoid of sacred chanting (japa) and meditation (dhyana) is sterile." **(XV.40)**

"One who chants mantras without taking precautions such as specific rituals is harassed by all sorts of obstacles, like a deer by a lion". **(XV.47)**

Here, *dhyana* or meditation relates to specific meditations of the deities and their forms, according to *sattvas, rajas* and *tamas* as per the individual and also their *dosha*. Mantras correspond to each of these also. Thus, as per Ayurveda, generic meditations cannot be given to people and must examine all other factors first, which also comes under the broader system of *Daivachikitsa* in *Charaka's* Ayurvedic system.

Asana:

Asana or posture refers to *Siddhasana* (perfected seated-position), the state by which all beings and enlightenment is gained and where the Yogi experiences no interruptions. This is known as the state of *Nididhyasana* in Vedanta and higher Yoga, where one becomes established in the Self by concentration or meditation and thus the seat here is establishment in meditation. That is the true meaning of *Asana* that grants all fruit of self-realisation and liberation (*moksha*).

This is also important. *Siddhasana*, the perfected pose that grant access to all of these higher powers by stilling the mind and body and purifying all subtle channels (*nadis*), is chief of all *Asanas* and others are of no sue when it is perfected and thus is the chief (*Hatha Yoga Pradipika*, I. 41-43).

A true Yogi or Yoga Teacher is thus one who can master this seated position and thereby brings about the fruits of all three *bandhas* (locks) simultaneously (*Mahabandha* - HYP, I.41.44) and thus by stilling the body, the mind is stilled and when the mind is stilled, all breaths can be stilled (thus pranayama) and by such, all senses are withdrawn (pratyahara takes place) it becomes single-pointed (ekagrata) and dharana takes place, through which one can access true meditation (dhyana) and enter into samadhi.

Likewise, *Kularnava Tantra* (17.62) states that *Asana* is called so as it yields *atmasiddhi* or perfection of the Self, prevents diseases and grants the nine *siddhis* or mystical powers of Yoga. As such, it also connects to *Siddhasana*.

The *Rig Veda* itself notes the importance of *Asana* as being stilled and the state where one attains the vision of the Gods, likening itself to *Kularnava Tantra's* description:

"He greatly meditates on the Devatas (Deities), where the immortals are seated."
-Rig Veda, IX.15.2

The term used here is *Asate* of which relates to an *Asana* or a seat also, having the same root. When meditating upon and also invoking the *Devata* in later Tantric *Pujas* or offerings, the deity is offered an *Asana* or seat. Here, it infers not only this, but also establishing the Deity in the heart in meditation in Yoga, as the *Atmaguru* or inner Guru and guide.

Here we also note that the deity *Varuna* has a firm-seat in the Rig Veda (VIII.41.9) as noted by the terms *'dhruvam sadah'* (fixed seat) where he becomes the ruler of the *sapta* or Seven, relating to the mastery over the seven worlds or *chakras*. This is also a clear reference to *Yoga* also; *'dhruva sada'* of *Varuna* here refers to his "fixed-seat", of

which is the true root and origin of *Patanjali's "sthira [sukham] asanam"* (*asana is that which is fixed and comfortable*) of which is also quite clear!
Another verse to the god *Indra* in the Rig Veda (III.35.4) states '*sthiram ratham sukham*' ("the chariot is still and comfortable").

The term *Ratha* here denotes the body and hence the body of *Indra* is *sthira and sukha*, meaning that it is still or fixed and comfortable. This is clear, direct reference to *asana* in relation to *Yoga* as being *sthira* and *sukham* or noting that the body should be so.

Another verse In the Rig Veda (I.121.12) states that the *horses of Vata (Pranas* or breaths*)* are again yoked by *Indra* - the "master of the senses" and the term *suyuja* is used, meaning "yoked well" or good. *Su* is also the root of course of *sukha* and refers to comfortable and alludes to the *sukhasana* and relates *asanas* or postures such as *siddhasana*, through which the *Vata* itself is brought under control or *prana* is stilled, since seated positions such as *sukhasana*, the most comfortable, help check *Vata* the best by being comfortable (*sukha*) and also seated (*asana*) - best for *Vata*. We can take much from this verse, by such terms alone!

On this note here, relating to incorrect *Asana* and the modern-day forceful movements of *vyayama-asanas* (exercise postures) in *Hatha-Yoga*, *Charaka* emphatically states (*Charaka, Chikitsa, IX.4*) that *Vishama-chesta* (difficult postures or movements) are also a cause for mental disorders or insanity and also makes a note here of foods etc. He also mentions not over-doing exercise and its uses (*Sutrasthana, VII.31-35*), especially those having psychological issues as anger, fears, *vata* disorders, old-age etc. This is a good lesson to be wary of today, relative to forceful *Hatha-Yoga* poses and diseases, especially *vata* types.

The warning here by *Charaka* is hence that if one's diet is not right and one is forcing movements, as well as being derisive towards the sacred Seers, priests etc. of Vedic traditions, insanity can be caused by any one of these, or meditational disorders, due to aggravating *sattvas* in the mind or heart (*Chikitsa,* IX.5-7). Today, we see Yoga groups and teachers violating all of these codes, which also suggests that in later life, or the next life, one will be born with psychological disorders as a result.

Before attempting *pranayama, Asana* or posture has to be first accomplished and perfected. This does not simply mean being able to perform all 84 *Asanas* as per *Hatha-Yoga*, but knowing their various *doshic* effects and mental effects, which make the body supple for sitting down for longer-periods in *siddhasana* and other seated-positions, which is the highest perfection of the limb of *asana*, such as being able to be seated, still (*sthira*) and be comfortable (*sukha*) without movement for long periods of time (as five to six hours) to that the mind-body is stilled so one can begin to perform *pranayama*.

Thus, before *asana*, the *yamas* and *niyamas* of Yoga must be first developed (*Hatha Yoga Pradipika, I.16.2-3*):

Ten Yamas of Hindu Yoga:

1. ***Ahimsa*** (non-violence towards any creature in either mind, body or speech)

2. **Satya** (truth-speaking for all beings through mind, body and speech)
3. **Asteya** (non-stealing through mind, body or speech)
4. **Brahmacharya** (celibacy or abstaining from sex in mind, body and speech)
5. **Kshama** (being able to endure both happiness and distress)
6. **Dhriti** (endurance or firmness of the mind during periods of gains or loss)
7. **Daya** (compassion towards creatures in all abodes)
8. **Arjava** (equanimity in mind, body and speech and avoiding forbidden actions)
9. **Mitahara** (moderate diet; taking only *sattvic* or sweet and oily foods)
10. **Shaucha** (cleanliness, both internally and externally)

Ten Niyamas of Hindu Yoga:

1. **Tapas** (austerities according to various rules and regulations of *sadhana*)
2. **Santosha** (contentment with whatever comes or we have)
3. **Astikya** (belief in actions as per the Vedas)
4. **Dana** (charity or giving without sense of reward such as monies, clothes etc. that are earned lawfully)
5. **Ishvara-pujana** (worship of the Deity with a pure mind, whether Vishnu, Shiva, Shakti, Ganesha etc.)
6. **Siddhanta** (study the sacred texts or Vedantic texts)
7. **Vakya-sravana** (listening to the sacred speeches; relating to commentaries)
8. **Hrimati** (modesty or shame and modesty as described in the Vedas)
9. **Japa** (chanting sacred mantras, either mentally or orally)
10. **Huta** (fire sacrifices)

Thus, only after perfection of these, can *Asana* be commenced. Hence, it takes several years, if not decades and sometimes lifetimes to accomplish these states and facets.

These differ slightly from other texts in Hindu systems, as the *Saivite Thirumandiram*, where *Hri* (modesty) is the first *Niyama* and *Siddhanta-shravana* is seen as one *Niyama* by itself, *Vrata* or sacred vows is added and *Huta* or sacrifices is indicated by the term *Tapas* or austerities. *Shandilya Upanishad* (I.1-2) also describes the Ten *Yamas* and Ten *Niyamas* and lists *Hri* and *Mati* as separate as shame (*hri*) as per Vedic injunctions and faith (*mati*) in those prescribed by the Vedas and *Vrata* as adhering to observances according to the Vedas.

Vakya-shravana relates to the stages of *sravana* (listening to the Guru about the transcendental states of Realisation) and then one moves into *manana* which is contemplating this truth internally and beginning to realise it. The final stage is *nididhyasana* where one is established in the Self and realises it (*Tripura Rahasya, XVII.65-67*).

Mitahara is also very important here also. It also falls under *shaucha* or purity of the system of *Patanjali's* Yoga, but from a traditional Hindu Yogic approach, it includes also adopting appropriate Ayurvedic diets according to seasons, climates (geographical changes), a person's age or stage of life, their sex (which has a bearing on overall constitution), digestive strengths, any diseases or genetic disorders (seen from the pulse, Astrological chart and examination of medical and family history). This also means adopting dietary regimes as per karmic implications astrologically, such as *gocharas* (planetary transits) and also *mahadashas* (planetary cycles) and their *bhuktis* (sub-planetary cycles under *mahhadasha*), by which regulation of diet and changes, implementation of some herbs etc. is required. This is a vast limb in itself.

Mitahara also relates to having *Sattvic* or pure foods according to these conditions, which sometimes have to be modified (for example, garlic and hing are considered *Tamasic* or dulling in Yoga, but may be required for medical purposes). Great Yogis also used formulas such as *Chyavanaprasha, Agastya Rasayana, Brahma Rasayana, Ashwagandha Rasayana, Bhringaraja, Triphala (for hair and eyes), Triphala Ghee (for eyes)* as well as those for joints as *Ashwagandha, Yogaraja and Mahayogarajaguggulu* and others as *Makardhwaja* and other mercurial and alchemical compounds for health and vitality, which come into dietary regimes here.

Ayurveda itself hence forms an integral part of the deeper Hindu Yoga system and all Gurus and Swamis traditionally trained in Yoga thus employ a range of sacred rituals along with Ayurveda, Vedic Astrology and their related rituals and practices into their Yoga regimes as integral parts. Today, the West and modern Yoga systems ignore these and few teachers have knowledge of Ayurveda itself, even at a basic level, let alone the use of rituals and Vedic astrology.

These should be kept in mind, considering the greater Yogic tradition also. Considering *Dhyana* or meditation, here, as per *Shankaracharya's* system, we thus have 31 levels to go beyond before we try and access meditation itself, which cannot be fast-tracked, as remember that Shankaracharya was dealing with Hindus living in India and knowing these systems themselves at a much earlier time in history and they were required then, even by advanced practitioners, let alone those today in the modern world that do not live in India, are not exposed to traditional Hindu-Vedic teachings and have no basis with which to develop these. Hence, integral Yoga systems are perhaps the most important aspect to bring forward for the future of mankind and their spiritual evolution, commencing with understanding first, these *Yamas* and *Niyamas* in greater depth beyond mere simplicity as an academic study alone.

Japa or chanting itself has mantras of three kinds, as per the three *gunas* of *sattvas, rajas* and *tamas*, according to their effects. Meditations also have such forms, according to the mind of the *sadhaka* or spiritual aspirant and also their own forms and have their own observances. As an example, for mantras,
the *Rishi* (Seer), *Devata* (deity), *Beeja* (seedmantra), *Chanda* (metre), *Viniyoga* (application), *Nyasa* (consecrations, such as common *Shadanga Nyasas* or full-body forms before using mantras), *Shakti* (power) etc. should all be known before using it. Some mantras also require these and special *Nyasas* in order to remove *shrapas* (curses) of deities and Seers to protect them, as they are enveloped in a mind of *kavacha* or armour that requires removal first.

Most mantras require energisation via these preliminary rituals (*purva-kriyas*) and then by chanting the mantra and offering into the sacred fire and such, but there are also other *Nyasas*, which can be considered as *Nyasangas* or "Limbs" under the aspect of *Nyasa* alone as also the science of *Chandas* or Vedic metres, which measures the syllables in any given mantras (itself one of the six *Vedangas* or auxiliary limbs of the Vedic teachings).

Such things as *Grahanyasa* (planetary consecrations), *Lokapalanyasas* (consecration of deities of directions), *Shivashakti-Nyasas* (consecration of the transcendental forces of *Shiva* and *Shakti*), *Pitha* (sacred places), *Achamana* (sacred sipping of water and cleansing after actions), *Bhumishodhana* (purification of the earth or abode), *Vighanivarana* (removal of obstacles), *Pushpashodhana* (purification of flowers), *Chittashodhana* (purification of the mind) are all part of the systems of *Nyasa* and *Puja* or sacred offerings and are examples of just some of the limbs. We mention there here simply to show the complexity of the deeper Hindu Yoga tradition, not simply its simplification. These form under the systems of *Japa* and *Ishvara-pujana* of traditional Hindu Yoga limbs or *Ishvara-pranidhana* in *Patanjali's* Yoga system.

Without these systems, going in for *asana* and other practices can be dangerous, as one's mind is not purified through these *Sattvic* methods to purify the mind at the deeper karmic level, such as *Charaka* also notes under insanity etc. and as conducive to a healthy mind. Without knowing these techniques also, meditation itself is also dangerous, as what meditations are best for one, as per their *doshic* type, diseases as also their own karmas can be dangerous. Generic meditations, like a generic medication hence can have side-effects if we do not consider the complete picture of the individual and take all factors into consideration first.

These can be seen as special *Yamas* and *Niyamas* of *Japa* itself and thus each have their own science in turn. These are also largely unknown to most people in the West practising Yoga and doing mantras and do not usually even know where mantras originated or their Seers, much less their pronunciation and deeper applications for energisation before use, and strict rules and regulations before performing them.

The Saivite text *Tirumantiram* (III.550) states that *kavacha* (protection), *nyasa* (consecration) and *mudra* (hand postures) are paths to reach the state of *Samadhi* or awakening the *Kundalini*-force itself, among with the *Yamas* and *Niyamas*. Thus, in integral Hindu Yoga systems, none of these is treated seperatly, but together as an integral part of the same Yoga itself, of which the Ten *Yamas* and *Niyamas* of Hindu Yoga also reveal.

People today using terms as *Ashtanga, Kundalini, Hatha, Bhakti, Jnana* etc. to describe their systems are thus using *Ekangavidya* (single-limbed wisdoms) rather than the integral Hindu systems, such as *Shankaracharya* and *Patanjali* both showed, which encompass all of these so-called "Yoga systems" as various levels along the path.

Bhakti or *Ishvara-pranidhana* (or *Ishvara-poojana*) is hence the basis that form the other levels of Yoga in the Integral or Vedic Raja-Yoga system, representing the various levels of *Vedanta* doctrines of *Dvaita* or duality, as one moves up the system, finally to *Advaita* or *Jnana*:

i. **Bhakti** (Dvaita)
ii.**Karma** (Visishadvaita)
iii.**Hatha-Kundalini** (Ishvaradvaita)
iv.**Jnana Yoga** (Advaita)

According to Vasistha Ganapati Muni (*Tattvanushasanam*), Yogas are:

Karmayoga: Doing good deeds without desire for rewards
Dhyanayoga: Meditation on mantras in the mind
Hathayoga: Control of breath (*vayu*)
Rajayoga: Controlling the *virritis* or waves of the mind
Jnanayoga: *Atmavichara* or Self-enquiry
Prapattiyoga (Bhakti-yoga): Offering the Self (to the Supreme)
Amritayoga: An integral approach of the above in attempt to purify
the *panchakoshas* (five bodily sheaths), fire of consciousness etc.

We must hence start at these base-levels of which *Ishvara-pranidhana* provides for us also. The *Vedic-Yoga* itself was mainly a *Bhakti-Yoga* (devotional Yoga) system with symbolism of *Tantric-Yoga* woven into its hymns, which makes it somewhat mystical in a sense or like a Tantric-text in poetry.

Relative to Yoga in Ayurveda and its application, these are very important here.

12 Sub-Yamas and Niyamas of Hatha-Yoga:

Along with the main *Yamas* and *Niyamas* listed above, we can classify some further types into these also in the tradition system of *Hatha-Yoga*, similar to those of *Shankaracharya* regarding his *Vedanta* system and others, such as his 15-Limb Yoga system.

These twelve *Upayamas* and *Niyamas* relate to the principles that can make or break us in Yoga and should also be given careful consideration in their own right:

There are Six Limbs that bring Success (*Prasiddhi*) and also Six Limbs that bring Destruction (*Vinashya*) in Yoga (*Hatha Yoga Pradipika, I.15-16*), relating more to these of diet and lifestyle that we should encourage and also avoid:

Six *Prasiddhi* or Successful Limbs are:

1. **Utsaha** (enthusiasm)
2. **Sahasa** (perseverance)
3. **Dhairya** (courage)
4. **Tattva-jnana** (Knowledge of 36 *tattvas* of Yoga or Yoga science)
5. **Nischaya** (unshakable determination)
6. **Janasanga-parityaga** (renouncing company of ordinary people; materialists)

Six *Vinashaya* or Destructive Limbs are:

1. **Atyahara** (overeating)
2. **Prayasa** (exertion)
3. **Prajalpa** (useless talking)
4. **Niyamgraha** (engaging in actions contrary to Yoga)
5. **Janasanga** (associating with people not conducive to Yoga; materialists)

6. *Laulyam* (unsteadiness)

To really understand these aspects of Yoga, we can hence begin to understand how disease can be manifested as a result of ignoring these *yamas* and *niyamas* in Ayurvedic Yoga, which are as important as the *dinacharyas* (daily routines) and *rtucharyas* (seasonal routines) employed in Ayurveda, as the basics behind preventing disease, as also avoiding incompatible food combinations etc.

By understanding these aspects here, the point is to show what *Charaka* denoted as causative factors for disease and the intricacies of these as explained in the greater Yoga system that is often not taught and these aspects not explained, thus causing great issues to people today practising these systems, opening up to powers and negative lower energies they have no understanding of nor control over, much less the prerequisites required for meditation etc. in Yoga and why these fundamentals as *yamas* and *niyamas* were first important to master.

IV: Understanding the Meaning of Prakriti:

Prakriti and *Vikriti* are often misunderstood in Ayurveda, as one's naturally-born constitution that doesn't alter and the deviating state of that respectively. However, more specifically they should be understood as not being of a *vata, pitta* or *kapha* type of person, or combination thereof, since the body is composed of all five *panchamahabhutas* respectively, though their variations may differ from the *dehika* or bodily or physical structure / appearance.

Here, the *Prakriti* is more specifically one's naturally or ingrained proneness or susceptibility to various diseases of *vata, pitta* and *kapha* or combinations thereof; it is also the natural state of *arogya* or health for these individuals also (one prone to *vata* disorders, keeping warm, having unctuous and warmer spices foods and not over-doing exercises and such, will be a healthier type). Here, the *Prakriti* of *arogya* types or healthy types, also known as *balya / vrishya* (strong) types, will be difficult to even assess according to the classical stereotyping of *vata, pitta* and *kapha* and their combinations, and thus should be taken here to represent simply the state of *arogya* or *sama prakriti* (equal state of the natural nature) wherein all three *doshas* are balanced. *Balya* or strength itself, says *Charaka*, is based upon three factors as *sahaja* (congenital), *kalaja* (based upon time or seasons etc. - exogenous factors) and *yuktija*, which is based upon diet and physical activity) - *Charaka Samhita, Sutrasthana, XI.36*. Here, we also remember the three main causes of diseases in *Ayurveda*, viz. *asatmya indriyartha samyoga* (misuse of the senses), *prajnaparadha* (misuse of the intellect), *parinama* (seasonal influences etc.), that alter the natural state or *Prakriti*. *Prajnaparadha* is the cause of both external disorders caused by elements, poisoning, wind and fire, as also psychological ones as jealousy (*irshya*), anxiety (*shoka*), fears (*bhaya*), anger (*krodha*) etc. (*ibid, Sutra,VII.*51-52).

This is further stated by *Charaka* (*ibid, Vimanasthana, VIII.95*) who uses the term "*dosha-prakriti*" to refer to the three *doshas*, but then refers to the state of *samadhatu* or the balanced state (the two terms being *dosha* - vitiation, implying a genetically disposed state and *sama-dhatu*, a constituent or equilibrium of these in their positive sense as a *dhatu*). He repeats this again after discussing the (predisposed) or *dosha-prakriti* dual-types (*ibid, Vimanasthana, VIII.100, VI.13-14. – they can only be of various "types" due to not having all dhatus / doshas equally – thus their features are shown by their 'aprakriti' or abnormal states alone*). The former (*vata, pitta, kapha*) are the unhealthy states that can suffer from various diseases in accordance with their proneness naturally (as per *dosha* predominant) and also *vikaras* as a result of other factors that aggravate the *doshas* as excessive intake of wrongful foods, incompatible foods, poisoning, seasonal changes and physical activity and foods or climates, injuries etc. which can differ from the *prakrita* (natural) diseases such a person faces normally.

The state of *vikriti* however should be taken as the state of vitiation, under which is easier to gauge, when a person is ill. Those having weaker constitutions, suffering from *vishamagni, tikshagni* or *mandagni* respectively will suffer from disorders of *vata, pitta* and *kapha* respectively as a result of the sensitivity to the *gunas* that aggravate any of these and their exposure, which is well known. *Roga* and *vikriti* then, are synonymous here, with the unhealthy state or deficiencies and excesses of any type; while the "natural state" (*Prakriti*) itself doesn't cause any harm, as a result of the sensitivity to say *laghu, shita, ruksha* etc. *gunas* of a person sensitive to *vata*, they will be more likely to suffer from these disorders (*vikiti*), as a result of the *gunas* inherit in them, which can become vitiated when a proper protocol for their palliation (*shamana*), such as *dinacharya, ritucharya, ahara, vihara* etc. are not properly implemented, which causes them to become disrupted.

Here also, *Ayurveda* details numerous *manasika vikaras* or vitiations of the mind (of the *tridosha* and beyond, as exogenous and other factors, viz. *rajas* and *tamas*), apart from the normal state of *manasika prakriti*, measured by a sixteen-fold model of psychic archetypes in *Ayurveda*. The *karmic prakriti* is yet another that is based upon past-life concerns related to *karma* of the individual that can be assessed via various charts and dictates the possible *prakriti* and also *vikaras* that individuals will have in any one given lifetime, and their prognosis.

Here, we must remember that a *vikriti* isn't solely of *vata, pitta* or *kapha*, but of their unions (*dvandva* - dual, *sannipata* - all three etc.), of which number sixty-two types alone in *Ayurveda* (*ibid, Sutrasthana, XVII.44*), in addition to *vikaras* arising from *Sushruta's* fourth *dosha* of *rakta* or blood. Here, the threefold are noted again (*ibid, Sutrasthana, XI.45*) as *nija* (innate), *agantuja* (external causes), *manasa* (psychic disturbances); *nija* is *shariradosha* (bodily *doshas*); *agantuja* is *bhuta* (external elements), *vishavayu* (toxic air or pollutants), *agni* (fire), *samprahara* (caused by wars, battles etc. or accidents) and *manasa* is that caused by unfulfilled *labha / alabha* (gains and losses). Here (*ibid, 46*) opposite therapies are given for the mind, as kind of placebo-therapies and keeping it happy and occupied elsewhere (hence meditation, mantra etc. to distract the mind from the unwholesome thoughts).

In addition to *dushya-nidanas* (vitiatable causes)
as *mamsaja* (muscular), *medaja* (fatty), *sahaja* (genetic), *karmaja* (karmic), *kshataja* (inj uries), *amaja* (internal toxins), *manasika* (psychic causes, viz. grief, anxiety, anger or other psychosomatic causes), *vishaja* (external poisoning or toxins), *krimija* (internal parasites and microbial infections, viruses) and so on as a result of *doshika* vitiation. These are all factors that cause *vikriti* or the movement away from the normal (*prakriti*) or *arogya* (healthy) state. Again, *Charaka* (ibid, *Sutrasthana, XVIII.48*) states that all three *doshas* exist in the body, either in their *prakrita* (natural) and *vikrita* (deviated, unnatural) states - hence again the question of a specific *Prakriti* stereotype per se, apart from one's inborn susceptibility, doesn't arise (i.e. *vatala, pittala* and *kaphaja* "body-types" - one assumes these are simply genetic abnormalities and weaker non *samadhatvika* types) - also. *Sutrasthana* VII.39-40, stating *sama* types don't have diseases, while the *vata, pitta* and *kapha* types suffer from diseases; the *dosha* here is the *dehaprakriti* or bodily constitution - meaning if outside the healthy state (*samadhatu prakriti*).

In conclusion then, with *Prakriti*, we must differentiate between calling them "mind-body" stereotypes, when they are more or less health-compromised constitutions listed with their sensitivities outside the healthier (*samadhatu*) types - here, the keys being *"dosha"* standing for vitiation or blemish and *dhatu* being a stable constituent as a positive true *Prakriti* itself in healthy form. While we can list *abalya / hina* (weak or poor), *madhyama* (moderate) and *balya / uttama* (strong, highest) types of the *doshika* variety of *dosha-Prakriti* (*Ashtanga Hridayam, Sutrasthana, I.9-10*), they must be differentiated from the *samadhatu* in terms and meanings as also examination, for the latter is a *balya* type which may have variables of build etc., but characteristics of *arogya* nonetheless, in addition to cancelling out the so-called *tridosha Prakriti* type, which doesn't fundamentally exist, but simply as a healthier state alone. Here again, the *Doshaprakriti* types are predisposed types and have no real "healthy" type among them, per se - but must be palliated through seasonal, daily and other routines to pacify them / help prevent and avoid diseases, contagious and otherwise. Whilst again the *Prakriti* cannot be altered, it does afford itself susceptibility due to its predispositions that we cannot ignore - being a "natural (*prakrita*)" course of disease - i.e. a *vata doshaprakriti* person means one that is predisposed to and more disorders caused by cold, rough, dry, light foods and climates as rheumatic complaints, dry skin, constipation, irritability, anxiety and insomnia etc. as a natural[1] (*prakrita*) course and being *aprakritiya* (unnatural) via other seasonal, climatic factors and changes, stages of life and times of the day, food and exercises contrary (a male in a *pitta* climate during *pitta* age and consuming too many spices would potentially cause an unnatural deviation from the norm, such as a *pitta-vikara* as excess anger, leading to skin rashes, liver issues or acid reflux etc.). An excessive aggravation (*prakopa*) of even the natural course can however produce an excess of the *dosha* which becomes harder to cure as a severe *vikara* (as a *vata* person that suffers from Parkinsonism or hemiplegia, for example, not milder diseases). *Dual-dosha prakritis* however are said to be *nindya* or blameworthy (*Ashtanga Hridaya, Sutrasthana, I.10*) – thus causing diseases.

The question of whether *prakriti* changes or not has been an ancient debate, but we can conclude that based on one's innate state of either stable health of the *dhatus* or a *samadhatva* type, or any of the genetically-predisposed *prakritis* (*doshaprakritis*, i.e. of *vata, pitta, kapha* and their combinations), such is in the negative. One remains predisposed toward such characteristics based upon the *gunas* and predominating gastric or *jatharagni* within them, for life. Note here, *Ayurveda* lists several diseases of congenital (*kulaja / sajaha*) disposition, including diabetes (*jata* – family and *bijadosha* – vitiation of the seed) causing incurability (*asadhyaja roga*) – *Charaka Samhita, Chikitsasthana, VI.57.*

While most people are *dvandvadosha* or dual-types (viz. *vata-pitta, vata-kapha, pitta-kapha*) and *vata* is almost always involved due to cold climates, foods, fast-paced lifestyles that influence the *prakriti* due to environmental factors not only for the embryo but also parents beforehand, *vata* is the cause of most diseases, which is why

---

[1] Note *Charaka Samhita, Vimanasthana, VI.15; 16-18*. Here, the *vikritis* are due to predisposed states of the non-*samadhatu* type that doesn't have equal tissues, hence of *vatala, pittaja, kaphaja* etc. types that are born predisposed to these respective diseases, which then become severe (as the same as the *prakriti*). In the modern world, due to bad diets, contradictory practices to *Ayurvedic* of ancient times, we often sadly find these are the case with patients, however, thus more complicating and difficult to treat that *vikritis* outside one's predominating type / predisposition. Our modern climate, as per *Ayurveda* (lifestyle and diet of parents, artificial drugs , refined and *tamasic* foods etc.), would also be seen as a stage for unusual vitiations, often of *vata* and *vata-dual prakritis* as most people are, regardless of their parents (*vata, vata-pitta, vata-kapha, pitta-vata, kapha-vata*). Many factors at the time of conception and mother's diet vitiate *vata* before birth, causing *vata prakriti* also – **see section on 'Rational Therapies and Genetics in Ayurveda'.**

the classics give such importance to *vata* and list the greater number of 80 diseases under it. As it moves other *doshas* it can also be (often) considered the primary cause of issues, as also most people having complaints being of *vata, vata-pitta, vata-kapha* varieties, with *pitta-kapha* not rare, but still predisposed to disorders of that kind, however with a stronger metabolism and enzyme function mixed with a stronger vitality (*ojas*), they can be easier to treat, often palliative, unless excessive deviation of the norms has been adopted by the individual.

Here, the original *Prakriti* based on the *doshas* is more connected with health-issues and temperament as in the TCM than the misguided "body type" view, beyond a matter of semantics, that exists in the modern *Ayurvedic* view and models, especially those presented in the west toda

V. Ayurvedic Types Beyond the Three Doshic Types:

While Ayurveda today commonly deals with three doshas alone, we should at this point however, note that Ayurveda's view of diseases is not limited to dosha-causes alone, as discussed. In fact, like *Sushruta* (*Sushruta, Sutrasthana*, XXI.16-17,25, *Sutrasthana*, I.25) *Charaka* also notes *Rakta or* blood (*Shonita*) as the fourth dosha in Ayurveda (*Charaka, Chikitsa*, V.27), which goes back to older schools of thought, yet as a *dosha*, it is seen more as an afflicted agent (*dushya*) than a *dosha* per se. These correspond to the four humors of Greek thought, viz. Black Bile (Vata), Yellow Bile (Pitta), Blood (*Rakta*) and Phlegm (Kapha), although the organs and elements are somewhat different and less sophisticated than the dosha model of Ayurveda. These form older schools of Ayurveda from *bahya* (outer) traditions of the Vedas and certain *Rishis*' views, going back to the time before the *Rig Veda* and the Ayurvedic Seers. The *tridosha* school is only one school alone, which became popular, as early as the *Rig Veda*.

Sushruta (*Sutra*, XXI.3, 16) also describes *Rakta* (*Shonita*) as the fourth *dosha* and also how it causes issues in the body and also in association with other *doshas* (29).*Sushruta* also further elaborates on other systems of Ayurveda that relate the different *Prakriti* types as arising from the *pancha-mahabhutas*, viz. *pavana* (vata), *dahana* (pitta or *agni*), *toya* (*jala* or kapha), *prithivi* (earth) with a large and stable or strong body and *nabha* (*akasha*) of a clean and long-life (*Sushruta, Sharira*, IV.80). This gives one more scope also, beyond even *rakta* as the fourth *dosha*, giving five main types and then various combinations of each of these.

Examination of the *mahabhutas* in man, which make up the *doshas* (as *dvandva mahabhutas* or dual-elements) and their degree in a person as also the twenty attributes or *gunas* is also a part of the deeper Ayuvedic examination of the *Prakriti* and disease-state that reflects astrological types which deal with these deeper aspects, physically and psychologically in traditional Ayurveda. Man himself is nothing but the expression of the five elements (*Sushruta, Sutra*, I.22).

We should examine these in the traditional scope also, for while the *tridosha* model is more useful than allopathy, it does not provide deeper insights into the exact elemental forces at play in the individual, which the *doshas* are mere expressions, not subtle forms of. Here also, the scope of *Prana, Tejas* and *Ojas* comes in, but of each also, formed by dual-aspects of *Vayu+Indra or Shabda+Sparsha, Agni+Apas or Rupa+Rasa* and *Soma+Prithivi or Rasa+Gandha* respectively.

Each individual has a predominance of one of the *mahabhutas* or combinations over others, which also give a more subtle and deeper view of their *Prakriti*. As an example, a *Vata* type with a strong digestion, memory and eyesight is a more *Vayu+Agni* type as a *Vata-Pitta* person, than calling them *Vata-Pitta* itself, which is a more generic way of categorising them according to four elements (two for Vata and two for Pitta), than assessing them individually.

Looking at the characteristics of the *Mahabhuta* types individually, we can assess them as follows, as per their elemental attributes (*Sushruta, Sharira, I. 20, I. 19, I.7*):

Akasha types will be sensitive to sound, ear disorders (as tinnitus and deafness) and feel spaced out. *Akasha* relates to *sattvas* or purity and hence there is a tendancy for such types to demand it from others. They relate to the deities of direction (*Disha*) and to *Agni* (Fire), relating to *Vak* or speech, relating to their element of *shaba* or sound and can become great mantrins or possessors of the power of mantra or speech. Of such types, there are *bala* (strong), *madhyama* (moderate) and *durbala* (weak) types accordingly. *Bala* types for example have strong hearing, sometimes even beyond the human norm as being able to hear inner divine sounds and the language of the Gods (Sanskrit) and ancient texts from upper worlds, while *durbala* types have very weak hearing and communication skills when their *sattvas* is more *tamasic*. More *sattvic* types can be masters of *shabda* or listening to the patient (as breathing, digestive sounds, joints etc.) and other deeper examinations in Ayurveda, as Vaidyas or Ayurvedic physicians and are able to diagnose through these deeper perceptions. Other types can heal through mantra, having the power of speech relating to their element.

Vayu types will be sensitive to touch, skin and nervous disorders, easily feel pains and feel light-headed at times. *Vayu* relates to *rajas* or action, which makes such types quite hyperactive at times (this is why *Vata* types having more *Vayu* than *Akasha* in their nature suffer from insomnia, anxiety etc.). They relate to deities *Vayu* (wind) and also *Indra* who rules the atmosphere and also presides over the hands (*hasta*), which also gives them a creative ability also, with their *rajas*. Of such types, there are *bala* (strong), *madhyama* (moderate) and *durbala* (weak) types accordingly. *Bala* types for example have strong tactile sensations, sometimes perceiving even subtle worlds, while *durbala* types have very weak sensations, going on to lack of sensations altogether, when *rajas* in them is less *sattvic* and more *tamasic*. More *sattvic* types can be masters of pulse diagnosis and other deeper examinations in Ayurveda, as Vaidyas or Ayurvedic physicians and are able to diagnose through these deeper perceptions. Other types can heal through touch (*sparshana*), having the power of *prana-shakti* via touch (as in pranic healing), relating to their element.

Agni (or *Taijasa*) types are sensitive to sights, colours, suffer more from eye disorders, feelings of hotness, strong digestions and glowing complexions, be angry and also brave. *Agni* has both *sattvas* and *rajas* in its nature and hence combines the properties of *akasha* and *vayu*, sensitivity and movement, but along with this, their fiery nature. They relate to the deities *Surya* (the Sun) and also *Prajapati* (creator) and can suffer from some *rajasic ahankara* or ego at times as a result, relating also to *upasta*, the uro-genital organ, making them somewhat sensitive to sexuality or having high passion and drive, as also infections in this region.

Of such types, there are *bala* (strong), *madhyama* (moderate) and *durbala* (weak) types accordingly. *Bala* types for example have strong eyesight and perception, sometimes even beyond the human norm, while *durbala* types have very weak eyesight to blindness, depending on how *sattvic* the *sattvic-rajas* is within them. More *sattvic* types can be masters of *rupa* or *drishti* - seeing and perceiving the diseases manifest on bodies as skin, the tongue and other deeper examinations in Ayurveda, as Vaidyas or Ayurvedic physicians and are able to diagnose through these deeper perceptions. Other types can heal through sight or looking at a person (their *yoga-drishti-shakti)*, having the power of sight relating to their element.

Apas types are sensitive to tastes and hence love foods and hold water in their bodies, are heavy in build and cold natured. Combined with other elements, they form dual-types such as the heavier water-holding *Vata* type, when combined with either *Akasha* or *Vayu*, or both (*Akashavayuava-jaleya* type, or *Vata* + *apas*). This is how *Sushruta's* mention of working with elemental types gives us a deeper scope to work with. *Apas* is *sattvas* and *tamas*, so brings in the lighter nature of *Akasha*, but also of the deeper dense aspect of *tamas*, relating to the earth. Hence, they have some movement, making them secondary *Vata* types. They relate to deities *Apas* (waters) and also *Mitra* (divine friend) and the anus (*payu*), relating to disorders there, or digestive issues related to their slow metabolism. Of such types, there are *bala* (strong), *madhyama* (moderate) and *durbala* (weak) types accordingly. *Bala* types for example have strong senses of taste perception, sometimes even beyond the human norm (not to mention their love of herbs and being around them), while *durbala* types have very weak to loss of smell altogether, depending on their level of *sattvic-tamas* within them, at the *sattvic* or *tamasic* scale respectively.More *sattvic* types can be masters of Ayurvedic diagnosis based on taste, as also perceive the deeper tastes and qualities (*gunas*) in herbs and substances and other deeper examinations in Ayurveda, as Vaidyas or Ayurvedic physicians and are able to diagnose through these deeper perceptions. Other types can heal through foods and herbs potentalised, having the power of taste relating to their element and hence able to empower these and infuse the *shakti* of dietary and herbal therapies better than other types when strong and perceptive.

Prithivi types are sensitive to smell and fragrances, have a large body and are heavy. They are the heavier or obese *Kapha* types that are more pure *Kapha*. *Prithivi* relates to *tamas* or inertia or darkness by itself, making them somewhat lethargic, unable to move or very slow in movements, whereas water types possess the movement of *akasha* or *sattvas*, making them more literally "fluid" in nature. *Prithivi* types tend to hold fat and gather more weight. Their sensitive smells also aid their cravings for foods in excess internally, which causes this stagnation. They relate to the deity of the earth, *Prithivi* and also *Vishnu*, the cosmic pervader, relating to the feet, the organs of movements and and stability, making them somewhat stable and complacent (stagnating) at times.Bala types for example have strong senses of smell, sometimes even beyond the human norm and able to smell fragrances in the upper worlds of the *Devas*, while *durbala* types have very weak to loss of smell altogether, depending on

their level of *tamas* within them, at the *sattvic* or *tamasic* scale
respectively. More *sattvic* types can be masters of Ayurvedic examination through smell
(*gandha*) and smelling the patient and their discharges (breath, urine, stool, sweat) and
other deeper examinations in Ayurveda, as Vaidyas or Ayurvedic physicians and able to
diagnose through these deeper perceptions. Other types can heal through aromas or
smells, having the power of smell relating to their element and hence can become
masters of these through essential oils, incense etc. and ability to heal through these.

In addition, we can itemise three more types, as per the *Samkhya* system, elaborates by
qualities in the texts:

Buddhi types, which are highly intellectual. Such types relate to *Brahma*, the creator
and share his characteristics. They are the more *Vata* and
analytical, *sattvic* and *Akasha* types, yet they are more primal in nature, more insightful
relating to sciences such as *Yoga, Ayurveda* and occult sciences as Tantra. They are
more *Rahu* types astrologically, with much insight of the head of the immortal serpent,
extending their insight beyond even *Ishvara* who controls the manifest world and
become great philosophers of the higher realms or deeply-inspiring philosophers of
traditions as *Shaivadvaita* etc. that go beyond the main *tattvas* or principles beyond the
world. Such types can make great psychologists in Ayurveda on the spiritual level,
especially relative to *bhutagraha* or seizures by astral spirits behind diseases and also
able to ascertain karmic causes behind diseases through esoteric methods as astrology
and divination.

Manas types, relating to the mind, are highly emotional, motherly and sensitive (like
Buddhist monks) and relate to the Moon (*Chandra*) in nature and qualities. They are the
more emotional and homely *Kapha* or *Apas* types, but more primal and original in
nature, caring for all beings throughout the cosmos and upholding *ahimsa* or non-
violence, somewhat like a *Bodhisattva*. They are lunar (*Chandra*) types astrologically,
kind, caring and also having long-life spans. Such types are able to diagnose diseases
based on a person's diet and are also very good are assessing the *ahara* or impressions,
physically and mentally a person brings into the body. Being more lunar, they also hold
deeper interest and wisdom of the *Soma* or *rasayana*, the science of rejuvenation and
longevity.

Ahankara types, which can be highly egotistical and also creative, relating
to *Ishvara* the cosmic controller. They are the regal *Pitta* or *Agni* types, but more primal,
original and creative beyond the physical sphere, as in types who can extend beyond the
literal into the scientific and spiritual insights and mysteries of the cosmos. They are
more *Ketu* types astrologically, the tail of the immortal serpent who penetrates into the
depths and mysteries of the cosmos, ruled by *ishvara*. Such types can also penetrate into
the depths of a person through deeper examination and diagnosis by looking at a person
and perceiving their past-life *samskaras* or karmic traits behind diseases at a more
subtle level and how to deal with them through rituals (*homa* etc.) and heal disease on
this level or through spiritual healing methods and modalities.

Each type also has specific psychological traits also.

Different categories of psyche and habits under each main *dosha* (Vata, Pitta and Kapha) are also mentioned in the *Samhitas*, relative to the sub-types of *doshas* (*Sushruta, Sharira, IV.66, 81, 86; Ashtanga Hridaya, Sharira, III. 89, 95, 103*): Vata-types - goat goyal, ox, rabbit, rat, camel, dog, culture, crow, donkey; Pitta-types -snake, owl, *gandharva*, *yaksha*, cat, monkey, tiger, beat and mongoose and Kapha - *Brahma, Rudra, Indra, Varuna*, lion, horse, elephant, cow, bull, red eagle and swan. Thus, the scope of three *doshas* beyond the normal three, especially relative to the mental types as per degrees of *sattvas, rajas* and *tamas* (as the elements or *mahabhutas* themselves are each attributed these), let alone the older scope and schools that saw four *doshas*, which included *Rakta*, which is an important aspect of Ayurveda.

The examination of the *gunas*, their percentages as well as *mahabhutas* and percentages in people is also part of Charaka and Sushruta's Ayurveda; the *doshas* are seen as but *dvandva* (dual) factors that occur as a result of these, but there may be any number of percentages of these in individuals beyond doshic concerns, which is why looking at these preliminary aspects is more specific, as is *Jyotisha*. As an example, a Mercurian type person is a more Vayu and Jala type; a specific Vata with secondary Kapha individual that has more psychic and emotional sensitivities due to higher Vayu *mahabhuta* (*sparshana* sensitivity and hence nervous disorders), but also secondary ability to retain Jala *mahabhuta* and hence put on weight by retaining water and kidney issues due to poor metabolism and kidney functioning. Such is an example that is often beyond the scope of the primary doshas, which are but indicators alone. Yet, *Rakta* as a separate dosha, as noted by *Charaka* and *Sushruta* also has its importance here in ancient systems.

What is more, these are also noted by Sushruta as relating to the pulse also. It hence appears that four *doshas* models existed in original forms of Ayurveda. While many argue that there is no mention of *Nadi-Pariksha* or pulse-examination in the classics. Charaka also knows of *Nadi-Pariksha*, although not elaborating upon it; he states the *nadis* are also within the bodily tissues along with the *dhamani* (arteries), *siras* (veins) and *srotas* (channels) of the body (*Charaka, Vimana, V.9*).

Sushruta further clarifies this under *sira* (veins) (*Sharira*, VII.8 - 28) notes of Vata, Pitta and Kapha in the veins of the body and their specific characteristics and diseases aggravations, also adding Rakta (blood) as the fourth dosha. *Sira* or veins he states, carry all the doshas (*Sharira*, VII.26) and he continues (verse 28) by stating the qualities of them; Vata is *aruna* (red) and filled with *vayu* (oxygen), *Pitta* is *nila* (blue) and *ushna* (hot) and Kapha is *gaura* (white), *sthira* (stable) and *shita* (cold) while *Rakta* (*asrig*) is *rohini* (crimson) and neither *shita* (cold) nor *ushna* (hot). *Sushruta* here describes the ancient system using four fingers for pulse-examination, perhaps employed in the *Shalyatantra* (surgical) school to which he belonged for identifying these four humors by proponents of his *Shastravidhi* (surgical-instrument) school.

Charaka and others note *Vishaja* (caused by poisons), *Kshataja* (caused by injuries), *Amaja* (caused by internal toxins) etc. types beyond the doshas, as also *Sahaja* (congenital types of diseases) and so forth also as causes; as with diabetes, we know there are some 20 types in Ayurveda, not simply of the three doshas alone.

This is where the modern Western "Ayurveda Programs" fail to address the deeper concerns as per traditional Ayurveda and their specific treatments, which remains superficialised at best. They often give students an incorrect and incomplete view and scope of the traditional Ayurveda mentioned in the classics, leaving it open to ridicule by western medical professionals, due to their emphasis of *daiva-vyapashraya* alone (and of that, a limited scope alone).

Some diseases such as *Rajayakshma* and *Ojas-kshaya* (deficiency of the immune system) are described by Charaka, much like modern AIDS. *Ojas-kshaya* is described as one being weak, mental agitation and disorders of the sense organs and caused by excess exercise, fasting, anxiety, rough foods or excessive loss of mucus, blood, semen etc. of the body (Charaka, Sutra, XVII.73-77). On this note also, Charaka also regards loss of semen (*shukra kshaya*) as a factor for causing diseases and death, due to it being the essence of food (*ahararasa*) in the body (Charaka, Nidana, VI.8-9). This is also the traditional view of protecting semen and *brahmacharya* (celibacy) to promote *balya* (strength) through retaining one's *ojas* (bodily vitality or immunity against disease). Such examples should be understood today to also really understand the Ayurvedic explanation and usefulness of practices such as celibacy in diseases, which are also ignored in India, as also in the West, where Ayurvedic practitioners continue to lead sexually-fulfilling lives and ignoring these ancient passages on preservation of bodily fluids. These therapies in themselves, while discussed, are not understood or implemented by practitioners and other treatments are still misunderstood further.

As an example piles today are Ayurveda in the West often miss traditional therapies such as *Kshara-sutra* (processed alkali threads) and the difficulty treating congenital hemorrhoids, fistula in ano etc. Then, as aforementioned, we have complex procedures from otoplasty and rhinoplasty that originated in Ayurveda to surgical correction of uterine prolapse. Yet, Panchakarma is popularised as the 'traditional' method West, which, albeit true from some perspectives was never, as we see, even in Charaka's opinion, the end-all solution and surgeons and their expertise were often recommended and patients referred to as per his own recommendations (i.e. *Shastrapatis* or Sushruta schools). Likewise, *Sharngadhara* for example lists 20 different types of possession-caused insanity, in addition to the doshas, Charaka and others add *vishavayu* (poisonous air or polluted air), which also relates to the causes of anxiety (*chittodvega*) and depression (*vishada*) of the modern-day, if we look deeply.

Charaka mentions three causes of diseases, viz. *Nija* (innate), *Agantuja* (exogenous) and *Manasika* (psychological) - Charaka, Sutra, XI.45. *Nija* is due to doshas; *Agantuja* is due to *bhutas* or elemental forces, which means poisoned air (*vishavayu*), fire (*agni*), *samprahara* (wounds due to accidents etc.) and *Manasika* due to desires and losses (*labhalabha*), mishaps (*anishta*) etc. The therapies he recommends (Charaka, Sutra, XI.46) are hence opposite therapies and those conducive to dharma.

Charaka also makes mention of *marmas* as vital organs (Charaka, Sutra, XI.48), namely *basti* (urinary bladder), *hridaya* (heart), *murdha* (head), *ashthi-sandha* (bone-joints) etc. Of course, the 107 Marmas first appear in the *Rig Veda Samhita* (X.97.1). On this, often ignored, is the great commentator and author of *Nirukta*, Yaskacharya who commentating on this verse, states *"Saptashatam purushya marmanam teshvena dadhatiti va" (Nirukta, Daivata Kanda,* 9.28). The 700 (*saptashatam*) mentioned by *Yaskacharya* here appears to denote the *Siras* or veins that run through the *marmas*, while *saptashatam* clearly are stated as marmas themselves in Vedic times, numbering 108. The Vedic verse mentions three *yugas* or ages of the gods in their connection, denoting symbolically the three doshas of Ayurveda that vitiate them. Thus their science was known and Charaka's own mention here, like his view of surgery also reveals that he considered them areas that when damaged, causing diseases (noting the *basti marma, hridaya marma* and *head marmas* as also those on joints as most important).

The other thing we should take note of are the *sahaja* or genetic factors, which should also be explained and also explained and understood via physical examination of '*kulaja ithihasa*' (genetic history), charts etc. and categorised as *karmaja* (or *atmaja*, karmic), *pitrija* (inherited from father's genes), *matrija* (from mother's genes), *matrija ahara* (mother's dietary impressions) and so forth to determine the exact methods of treatments, spiritual and also exoteric or rational. It is also important that the general public and also practitioners in the West understand the place of genetics and congenital diseases in Ayurveda and their formation, as also compared to modern-science to also bring Ayurveda's validity or credence into the modern world also, which also helps in general acceptance of its therapies or modalities by understanding it properly, not simply in the pasteurised New Age fashion, which does more harm than good. Ayurveda's view of subtle factors behind congenital as karmic, the effects of foods, diet and lifestyle are also important factors to consider here and bring into the world, along with surgery, internal detoxification etc. as mentioned by *Charaka* and others.

For example, *Charaka (Chikitsasthana, IX.96)* also states that insanity can be avoided if one abstains from eating meats and wines or impure diets etc. and hence these substances are seen as causative factors (*nidanas*) of various kinds of insanity. The commentator on *Charaka Samhita, Chakrapanidatta* (commentating on *Sutrasthana, I.54)* also states that *prajaparadha* or perversion of the intellect causes one to commit bad deeds (karmas). Taking of impure foods (*ashuchi-bhojana*), insulting teachers and learned people (*pradharshana* - attacking, *devagurudvijana* - gods, Gurus and twice-born, i.e. *Brahmins*), mental shock or fear (*bhaya*), excitement (*harsha*) and irregular or forced /exertion of bodily movements (*vishama ca cheshta* i.e. as in *Hatha-Yoga vyayamas* or exercises) cause insanity *(Charaka, Chikitsa,* IX.4-5) This causes the bodily biological humours to become aggravated and dulls the truth-perception or reality of the person (*sattvas*) in the heart (of the mind), enter the mental-channels (*manovahani*) and derange the mind of the person *(Charaka, Chikitsasthana, IX.4-5).* This also means taking incompatible foods such as milk with seafoods, artificial poisons or emotions such as anger (*krodha*), which can damage the mind, according to *Chakrapani,* the commentator on Charaka Samhita. Insanity is the delusion (*bhrama*) of the *buddhi* (intellect), *manasa* (emotional mind) and *smriti* (memory) and of two types, *agantuja* (external) and *nija* (internal), but classified as five types, viz. *Vataja, Pittaja, Kaphaja, Sannipataja* (*tridosha*) and *Karmaja* (classified under exogenous) - *Charaka, Chikitsa*, IX.8-16.

On this note, *Sushruta* also notes of six types, viz. *Vataja, Pittaja, Kaphaja, Sannipataja, Manasa Dukha* (unhappiness in the mind, caused by threats, loss of wealth, injuries etc.) and *Vishaja* (poisons), also known as *Mada* (intoxication) - *Sushruta, Uttara,* LXII.4-5, which produces *moha* (delusion), *dvega* (confusion of the mind) etc. (*Uttara,*LXII.6-7).

This is all caused by abnormalities (or toxins or intoxication, *mada*) in the upper paths of the mind (*Uttara*, LXII.3), what we can call chemical imbalances of the mind also. For *shoka* (grief) caused, counselling is implied, by removing the grief and hence *chitta-prasadana* (purification of the subtle mind or *Chitta - Uttara*, LXII.34-35). This would also include therapies such as *jyotisha* (astrology) to help reduce past-karmic impressions causing toxins in the *chitta* etc. as *homa* etc. under *Daiva-vyapashraya* mentioned earlier and helping bring more *sattvas* or equilibrium to the mind, freed from these toxic impressions or chemical imbalances of the mind.

On this note also, *Sushruta* (*Sutrasthana, XIX. 3*) mentions *Vastu* or the science of *Vastu-shastra* or Indian Feng Shui when selecting a dwelling for wounded people, where he commences stating that sacred hymns be chanted, special fumigation done etc. to ward off negative astral entities and the physical parasites and bacteria that can be caused as a result of them. This is to ensure the surroundings are also *sattvic* for the mind and body also; the same were true of certain *rasayana* or rejuvenation therapies. *Vastu* itself, relating to *jyotisha* and Ayurveda then is an integral part, as is Yoga.

Sattvas (purity, truth, and perception), *rajas* (passion, action, agitation) and *tamas* (darkness, ignorance, delusion) are the three functions that affect the mind. Ayurveda knows sixteen varieties of these types that afflict the mind, according to their gradients of each (seven *sattvic* sub-types, six *rajasic* sub-types and three *tamasic* sub-types), although several more divisions exist.

This is something modern allopathic medicine also does not consider, nor does it consider the effects of foods, herbs and substances and their effect on (a) the doshas and their aggravation in diseases and vital organs and (b) the effect of them causing *malas* (wastes) in the mental channels, bringing about chemical imbalances in the brain. As per the dietary therapies of Ayurveda alone then and its depth of understanding substances overall, it is far ahead of modern medicine, which is yet to investigate these effects or causative effects behind diseases (as it is a factor ignored). As an example, as per Ayurveda, foods such as meats, excessive spices, heavy foods, canned or preserved foods, pickles etc. can aggravate the mind and bring about chemical changes in the mind that can cause a variety of mental disorders from anxiety to Schizophrenia and can aggravate these conditions. Restoring normality and equilibrium to the mind (*sattvas*) is brought about by sattvic diets and foods, as also specific herbs that also help to impart this and improve brain activity (as *Brahmi -* Barcopa monniera, *Gotu Kula -* Centella asiatica etc.). Several specific formulas as *Saraswata Churna* [4], *Kalyanaka Ghrita, Brahma Ghrita, Manasamitra Gudika* [5] etc. also exist in Ayurveda to improve brain activity, clear mental channels of toxic chemical blockages or wastes behind these issues and restore normality to the mind and body. While Charaka mentions many of these, as other authors, the system is much older.

As an example, there are cases of ancient Ayurvedic remedies, such as *madhu* (honey) for diabetics, said to reduce blood-sugar levels etc. in Kapha types (diabetes being a Kapha disorder), which modern studies have also revealed [6].

VI. Antiquity of Ayurveda and Surgery in the Vedas:

We can defend the history of Ayurveda and various aspects of it, not simply limited to Charaka, who was one of the final redactors of the ancient tradition.

Ayurveda itself traces its origin back to the Vedic deities, the *Ashwins* and Seers such as *Atreya* and *Bharadvaja* as well as to the Kings of Kashi (modern-day Varanasi or Benares) such as the *Divodasa* lineages. We see these names in the Rig Veda, the oldest of texts and also the healing feats of deities such as the *Ashwins* and also deities such as *Rudra* and *Soma* are lauded as divine doctors and associated with herbs (*bheshaja*). The science of Ayurveda then goes back to Vedic times as a branch of this knowledge, as also does Tantra itself.

Tantric Ayurveda itself is seen in the *Rig Veda* and *Atharva Veda*, where special mantras, charms etc. are used in healing. The *Krishna Yajurveda* is also the major basis of later *Shaivite* traditions in India, through which *Tantric Ayurveda* derives.

Classics also mention various *Sampradayas* or schools of Ayurveda, at the time of *Agnivesha*, the Guru and teacher of *Charaka* and *Agnivesha's* own Guru, *Purnavasu Atreya (Charaka Samhita, Sutrasthana,* XXVI.3)-:

-**Shakunta**
-**Mudgala**
-**Kushika**
-**Bharadvaja**
-**Videha sampradaya**
-**Dhamargava**
-**Bahlika sampradaya**
-**Atreya**

Atreya himself was from the *Bharadvaja* lineage, but appears to represent another school of it. His students also formed individual schools of their own also, based on his own teachings (*Charaka, Sutrasthana,* I.30-31): *Bhela, Jatukarna, Parashara, Harita and Ksharapani.* Thus, of these several lineages, the *Charaka* lineage of *Agnivesha* became the most famous - despite the various other lineages existing at a former time with their own views - which mention various lineages describing the numbers of tastes (*rasas*) in Ayurveda, as per each of these schools.

Likewise, Charaka Samhita (Chikitsa, XXVI.122-124) describes ninety-six eye diseases as per the system of *Karala*, yet others such as the systems of *Videha* (seventy-six) and *Satyaki* (eighty) are known to have existed also as per the commentator, *Chakrapanidatta.* Similarly, *Charaka* (*Sutra*, XXVI.64-65) states some systems of Ayurveda state there are eight forms of *virya* or potency of herbs (i.e. soft, sharp, heavy, light, unctuous, rough, hot and cold), which others state only two (i.e. *ushna*, hot and *shita* cold). Thus, even what we deem today as "Traditional Ayurveda" had itself, several ancient diverse systems, of which the current (of *Charaka* and *Sushruta*) have come down to us in redacted forms. Even the

Dhanvantari-Sushruta school of surgery appears as one line alone of the ancient system going back to the Ashwins.

Many things in modern Ayurveda we also ignore from the classics; Charaka states brushing the teeth with twigs twice daily, along with scraping the tongue with scrapers made from gold, silver, copper, tin or brass, chewing of cloves, betal, camphor or cardamom etc. and oil-pulling to prevent diseases of the teeth and gums (*Charaka*, *Sutra*, V.71-80); yet in the Western world, these have only recently been implemented and of that, namely toothbrushes. It shows the levels of hygiene in ancient India compared to the West from ancient times.

Other older lineages include that of *Bhargavas* such as *Chyavana*, famous for the formula *Chyavanaprasha* and connected to the original science of *rasayana* or rejuvenation. *(Rig Veda, I.116.10, I.117.13, I.118.6, V.74.5, VIII.68.6, VIII.71.5X.39.4, X.61.2)*. The original Seer *Atri* of the *Atreya* lineage is also connected to the original teachings of the *Ashwins* (*Rig Veda,* I.183.5, V.73.6-7 etc.) as having been saved by them.

We also have the *Kashi* school of *Sri Dhanvantari* through *Sushrutacharya*, which appears to have been a surgical school associated with oral traditions of facial reconstruction with the epithet *"Sushruta"* being applied to them (*su-shruta* = "one who hears well"). This is generally also the *Vishwamitra* lineage. *Vishwamitra Rishi* himself in the Upanishads is connected to hearing also, via the ear (right ear, *Brihadaranyaka Upanishad,* II.2.4). This also relates to the Vedic *shruti* (heard) tradition, which would have included surgery, as per *Sushruta* (*Sutrasthana,* I.16-20). This is noted in the *Rig Veda* itself, relative to ENT reconstructions and the *Ashwin* gods it came from (Rig Veda: II.39.6). On this note, tradition tells us (*as Dalhana,* commentator on *Sushruta Samhita*) that there was an older *Vriddha Sushruta* or *Saushruta Samhita,* of which the present is a redacted form. *The* grammarian *Panini* also notes traditions of *Sushruta* or *Saushruta Parthiva,* which also reveals an ancient tradition dating back before *Sushruta* of the *Samhita,* going back to Vedic times and hence to the *Ashwins*. There also existed the longer *Ashwini Samhita* of the *Ashwins,* which details advanced surgery such as head transplants (*Sushruta Samhita, Sutrasthana, I.17)*, organ and limb transplants or cybernetics, as is revealed in the hymns of the *Rig Veda* on this note.

At around 600BCE, *Jeevaka*, the Buddha's surgeon used a special gemstone (called *sarvabhutaprasadana*: that which pacifies all elements) which reflected the inside of a patient's body, to see the internal condition before he operated (like an X-Ray). *Jeevaka* is known to have successfully employed anesthesia, removed brain-tumours surgically and also fix twisted bowels.

The text "*Bhoja-prabandha*" of about 980AD deals with the life of the great King *Raja Bhoja*. In it, it was stated he was suffering from a brain tumour and two Ayurvedic surgeons were brought to him. Using a special drug, they made him unconscious, opened his skull, took out the tumour and then restored the skull with special Ayurvedic techniques and with another medicine, brought him back to consciousness. Hence, not only was brain surgery well-known in Ayurveda, but also medicines that induced comas and reversed the effects for complex operations also. After this, Raja *Bhoja* was fine and lead a normal life, free from any complications and this also shows the level of skill and depth of scope in traditional Ayurveda.

Charaka (Chikitsasthana, I.4.39-51) also mentions the advanced surgery of the *Ashwins*, echoed in the *Rig Veda* also, of the *Ashwins* replacing teeth and eyes of the deities also; eye transplants are also noted in *Rig Veda* (I.116.16, I.117.17-18) with successful outcome, by which *Rjrashva* was able to see again. Whether symbolic or not, that *Sushruta* and *Charaka* both praise them and their skill in *shalyatantra* or surgery to perform these feats and *Sushruta* praising surgery as originating from them, as also later techniques as previously described, and *Sushruta's* own techniques, which were advanced as plastic surgery, only a few hundred years old in the West due to originating from his system, makes us also realise the depth and scope of ancient Ayurvedic physicians, who performed transplants and techniques far beyond even today's modern surgical scope that has re-evolved from *Sushruta*!

The *Rishis* all appear to have learnt the science from *Indra* (Lord Shiva) himself however, which is also why we get so many lineages and why the Tantric lineages claim to descend from Shiva also as the others. *Indra* was the ancient name for Shiva and hence appears in the classics. Later Ayurvedic Seers such as *Madhavacharya* and *Sarngadhara* also revere Shiva as the master of Ayurveda for this reason, as the older classics of *Sushruta* and *Charaka* mention Indra.

The great seer *Kakshivan* in the Vedas who is associated with the *Ashwin* gods of healing for example (*Rig Veda*, VIII.9.10, X.143.1), is also son of Seer *Dirghatamas* like the historical *Dhanwantari* and likewise associated with Indra, as his earthly form (*Rig Veda*. IV.26.1). Indra also gives *Kasihivan* his wife, *Vrichaya* (I.51.13). *Kakshivan* also praises the *Ashwins* (*stotaram, Rig Veda.* I.112.11) and they also teach him (*Rig Veda*, I.116.7). Likewise, Indra also asks the deity *Dhanvantari* himself to take avatar in the world of men and learns Ayurveda from him according to *Bhavamishra* in his *Bhavaprakasha* on the origin of Ayurveda. The Seer *Bhavamishra* also places *Charaka* himself as an avatar or incarnation of the god Vishnu, like *Dhanvantari*. In a hymn to the deity *Brahmanaspati*, *Kakshivan* is also lauded in the *Rig Veda* (I.18.2), where the deity is lauded as a remover of disease (*amivaha, Rig Veda, I.18.3*).

Later Ayurveda and Yoga has 72,000 *Nadis*, which run through the body. These 72,000 *Nadis* are actually mentioned of in the *Rig Veda* (VIII.46.22) symbolically as 70,000 Cattle and 2000 Camels. The next verse (23) states that the horses with long tails turn the Chakra of the Chariot or wheel of the body, which is exactly what the Nadis do - revolve around the Seven Chakras or Energy-centres in the body, showing in what context is implied here. Verse 26 of the same also notes the 21 Chakras (thrice seven times) with 70 horses.

Of these, 1000 are said to be '*syava*' or brown or black in hue, relating to Vata and ten red ones (*rusha*) in three locations, relating to Pitta. Of these, the '*syava*' or brown or black ones (Vata) makes the rim (*nemi*) turn – relating to circulation of Vayu in the body making the *doshas* move. Vata and Pitta are mentioned here, since they both are the more important; Vata creating most diseases and Pitta secondary. Kapha produces the least disorders. These are also connected to the knowledge of taking the *nadi* or pulse as mentioned earlier, relative to *Sushruta's* mentioning the *doshas* in the *siras* or veins. *Rig Veda*. IX.32.3 also notes that *Soma* (Kapha) is like a swan (*hamsa*), which refers to the later *hamsa-gati* (swan-like movement).

In the *Brihadaranyaka Upanishad* (II.1.19) the Seer *Yajnavalkya* also mentions the 72,000 *nadis*. In IV.3.20, he describes their colours as white, brown, blue, green and red, and states they are like a hair split 1000 times, showing how subtle they are, relating to the several *nadis* in later Yogic lore, of which form the even more subtle aspect of *Nadi Pariksha* in Yoga, from which Ayurveda derives the system. This all describes the very (even more ancient) refined Pulse science of ancient India of the primordial Rishis. What we have today in Ayurveda is quite a limited concept. Moreover, relating to *nadis* and *chakras*, it also reveals from traditional texts, how minute or atomic in size they actually are and hence are not able to be felt or perceived by one and all. For this reason, *Kanada*, the ancient Vedic atomist and founder of *Vaisheshika* or atomic-phsyics, is also an ancient authority on the pulse as well.

Rig Veda, IV.31.1-2 mentions a *ratha* or chariot that was made without reins or horses, with three wheels that remains in movement or action (*rajas*; term used is *rajah* – firmament etc. which relates to *rajas*). This refers to the three locations of the three fingers on the *Nadi* or pulse. It also relates it to being created from *manas* (mind) and related to meditation or thought (*dhyaya*, relating to *dhya* – meditation or contemplation).

The Three Divine-medicines (*divya-bheshaja*) and Three Earthly Medicines (*tri-parthava*) are described as given by the *Ashwins*, relating to the Three Doshas (*tri-dhatu*) and preserving or protecting them (*sharma*), which relates to Spiritual and Herbal therapies in Vedic times for mitigating the Three Doshas. (I.34.6), as also the Three doshas along with Vata's importance, being related to Atman or the Soul (as the concept of *Prana*).

The Seer *Agastya* of southern India is also an authority on Ayurveda, especially *Rasa Shastra* or the science of alchemy. In the Vedas, he is also associated with deity *Indra* and the *Maruts* in the Rig Veda (I.170.3) which later become the basis of later Tantric masters or *Nathas* and *Siddhas*. In another hymn in the *Rig Veda* (I.117.11), *Agastya* is said to have invoked the *Ashwins* to that queen *Vishpala* could have her prosthetic leg.

The science of alchemy also derives from the older traditions in the Rig Veda and is connected to the Seer *Chyavana* and the *Bhargavas* as previously mentioned. The great alchemist, *Nagarjuna* (c.200AD) was said to have originally been a Brahmin before becoming a Buddhist and appears to have been connected to the older *Shaivite-Vedic* tradition of alchemy also and in older texts as the *Artha Shastra* (c.400BCE), use of Mercury etc. are also mentioned. *Ksharas* or caustic alkalis are commonly mentioned in the classical texts, as are the properties of various metals.

Bhasmas or use of gold ash and those of precious stones are also mentioned by *Charaka* and *Sushruta* in various places.

Sushruta (*Uttarasthana*, XXXXV. mentions *parada* (mercury) and *churnaka* (limestone), *manashila* (arsenic sulphide) etc. in a preparation for infant insanity or possession and again mentions *parada* (mercury) in relation to a preparation for skin diseases (*Chikitsasthana,* XXV.39). He also mentions the therepeutic properties of metals and gemstones (*Sutrasthana*, XLVI.326-330). Thus, the science of alchemy was well-established by his time, at least 600BCE, if we look at the redacted versions (which must have been finalised prior to the Buddha).

In the *Rig Vedic* hymn to *Rudra-Soma* as the Gods of Healing (VI.74.1), we find reference to the *Sapta-ratna* or seven gemstones, that relate to the seven main planets ruled by the Sun (or *Adityas*) - those for the Sun (ruby), Moon (pearl), Mars (red coral), Mercury (emerald), Jupiter (yellow sapphire), Venus (diamond) and Saturn (sapphire), which also notes their ancient therapeutic use, relating to the planets, as also in the form of medicated ash (*bhasma*) etc.

Charaka (*Chikitsasthana*, I.3.5-23, I.3.46-47, I.4.13-26) mentions various *rasayana* or rejuvenation formulas containing heavy metals, such as *loha* (iron) as in his recipe for *Lauhadi Rasayana*. One certain *Rasayana* formula ascribed to *Indra* (*Chikitsa, I.4.13-26*) also mentions *hema* (gold), *tamra* (copper), *ayas* (iron), *sphatika* (quartz crystal), *mukta* (pearl), *vaidurya* (cat's eye), *shankha* (conch-shell) and *rajata* (silver) *churna* (powers, i.e. *bhasmas* or medicated ash) as in later times. *Charaka* in older portions of *Sutrasthana* (I.70) also mentions *suvarna* (gold), *pancha loha* (five irons or metals - viz, silver, copper, iron, lead and tin) and their arsenic sulphides (*manashila*), gems (*mani*), salts (*lavana*), *gairika* (haematite), *anjana* (galena) etc.

The Rig Veda mentions the metallic leg of *Vishpala* cast by the *Ashwin*-Gods (I.116.15). Interestingly, this is the same hymn that also mentions Rishi Agastya, formally mentioned also relating to the Ashwins and who is associated in southern India with the traditions of r*asa-shastra* or alchemy also! The *Atharva Veda* (II, 19.26) also mentions gold amulets relating to long-life. Pearl, lead etc. are also mentioned as amulets in the *Atharva Veda* also. The term aya appears commonly in the Rig Veda as a generic term for metal also, which is interpreted accordingly, like other Sanskrit terms as per various sampradayas or lineages of Sanskrit etymology (of which, numerous schools exist). The deity *Soma* in the Vedas is also a deity associated with immortality (*amrita*) and in later times also denotes *ojas* (vitality), *aushadhi* (herbs) and other formulas or *rasayanas* that prolong life also, including *parada* or mercury.

Rudra, a form of Shiva as the divine healer is lauded as having a thousand (sahasra) medicines (bheshaja) in the Rig Veda (VIII.46.3), which also relate to *Soma* as the sahasrarapadma-chakra or thousand-petalled lotus, which in later times, as the Crown of the head is the seat of *Soma* as immortality and relates to mercury. Mercury is also called *rasa*, which also means "taste" in Sanskrit, relating to the inner-taste or sweet-taste of the *Soma*-juice which when rains down provides immortality, through the process of *khechari-mudra,* where the tongue is positioned at the back of the mouth.

This is also referred to as "honey/sweet-tongued' (*madhu-jihva*) in many other Vedic verses also, where the inner *Soma*-juice is tasted by the Yoga as the immortal nectar (*amrita*) that rains down when pierced by the tongue:

"Exhaust-less and with a sweet-tongue (madhujihva), they have sent their voices down in unison, in the Shining region that flows in a Thousand streams (thousand petals)."
-Rig Veda,IX.73.4

Interestingly, the same madhu or sweet-science, relating to science of rasa or taste and later Mercury. The Seer *Dadhyach* in the Vedas is also transformed by the physician-gods, the *Ashwins* and is son of the seer *Atharvan*, who is noted as having wisdom of the later *Atharvaveda*, from which Ayurveda itself arose. They restore his head to him, but as they do with others, also teach him the science of *Soma* (RV.I.119.9) -
Soma being *amrita* or immortality and including alchemy in Vedic thought or honey (madhu; also meaning "sweet" and primary of the six later *rasas* or tastes in Ayurveda). *Dadhyach* as noted personifies *Indra's Vajra* or thunderbolt, whose head is cut off in order to reveal the *Soma* or nectar of immortality (RV.I.134.13-15). *Dadhyach* thus also grants the *amrita* or immortal *Soma* and is lord of *Soma* (RV.IX.108.4), thus connected to the science of *rasayana* or rejuvenation and *rasa-shastra* or alchemy and hence its ancient origins from Vedic times.

Mercury (*parada* or *rasa*) is also known by the synonyms of *Shiva* (*Indra*) himself, such as *trinetra* (three-eyed), *rasendra* (king of tastes) etc. Like *Soma*, Mercury is also related to the colour *shukra* or white and also semen, and as such is said to be the semen of Lord Shiva that fell upon the earth. Soma itself is also commonly lauded as *shukra* (meaning both 'effulgent' and 'semen') in the *Rig Veda* (IX.54.1) and is likewise also white (*shweta*, Rig Veda, IX.74.7, 74.8) and thus also stands for Mercury also in the Vedas.

This all reveals the antiquity of these traditions in Ayurveda and the scope of the older Ayurveda. As we see, things from *marmas* to the ancient term *Sushruta* in the Vedic texts stood for surgeons etc. and are extremely ancient. What we have from the extent Ayurveda today is but a smaller and condensed, perhaps *Raja* or royal tradition by which employs the *tridosha* system and others, but replaced, in later times, the much older Ayurveda, which also was included *Pashavayurveda* (Veterinary science) and *Vriskhayurveda* (Botany), which themselves had innumerable branches and should not be forgotten by the mere human system today.

Charaka Samhita (*Siddhisthana, XI*.19-26) describes the various enemas and the use of herbal decoctions for elephants, camels, cows, horses, sheep and goats; similarly, *Sutrasthana* (I.92-113) mentions various therapeutic effects of the urine and milk of various animals and also credits goat-herds, shepherds, cow-herds etc. as possessing the knowledge of name and forms of various herbs only (which suggests also a limited, but localised knowledge of *Vrikshayurveda*). *Charaka* (*Sutrasthana,*I.72-73) also mentions four types of vegetable origins for herbal medicines; *Vanaspati* (trees), *Virudha* (climbers), *Vanaspatya* (shrubs) and *Oshadhi* (herbs).

VI: The Issue of Satmya (Suitability) in Ayurveda:

Today, Ayurveda is seen as being a predominantly vegan or vegetarian system resting on *ahimsa* of non-violence. While this is important, we must first take note of *dehika ahimsa* or non-violence relative to our own bodies, which requires eating suitable foods as per our diseases, constitutions and also relative to genetic and social *satmya* or suitability. Here, there is a difference between taking meats (which were traditionally ritualistically sacrificed and taken when needed) for certain purposes as per their requirement and mercilessly killing in excess as today's abattoirs.

According to the classical texts, we must examine and treat people according to their cultural *satmya* or suitability of *ahara* or accustomed foods and intake relative to their *desha* or location and climate - which isn't the same as, or even across India!

On *satyma*, Sushruta (*sutrasthana*, XXXV.39-40) notes that various substances and foods that don't cause any vitiation, despite their contrary nature to one's biological constitution, the region, season and even exercise regimes, are suitable, as one becomes accustomed to such. Good examples are royal families that habitually take alcohol and meats as also rich foods and yet don't suffer from diseases of excesses due to suitability of these through various generations - compared to non-aristocrats that could not historically afford such and being not used to these, can suffer from excesses when taking such.

Samtya or suitability is also mentioned by *Charaka* in greater detail (*Charaka Samhita, Chikitsa*, XXX, 315-19), especially relative to Chinese, Persians, Central Asians and Greeks habitually eating meats and taking wine and thus becoming accustomed to them, and of southern Indians with lighter foods as tubers, roots and fruits and variations such as suitability of fish as in eastern India (Bengal etc.); in the Sindhi region, the liberal use of milk-products is noted and grains as wheat and barley with milk in the central region of India, and that despite being unhealthy, such accustomed or suitable (*satmya*) foods should be given to these patients along with medicines for better health, rather than changing it and forcing a localised diet upon them!

This is mentioned in *Charaka* in ancient times – yet today, we see the same people as the Europeans and others (Greeks and Persians mentioned in the classics along with Chinese) being administered a south-Indian style vegetarian staple along with various herbs for their conditions, opposed to their (local and genetic) suitable foods, when even a native Indian of Bengal or Sindh wouldn't be customised to such diets!
In more recent times, the south-Indian vegetarian staple that *Charaka* mentions (suitable to the *pittogenic* climate of south Indian Brahmins due to it being hot and damp or humid), has come to replace many dietary regimes in India as "*sattvic*", due to the influence of historical *acharyas* or teachers coming from the south in ancient times as south-Indian Brahmins (*Shankaracharya, Ramanuja, Vallabhacharya, Nimbarkacharya, Madhavacharya*) and modern Gurus coming from there, including *Sri Ramana Maharishi, Satya Sai Baba, Bhagavan Nityananda, Swami Sivananda* etc. Yet, these diets are not suitable to non-*pitta* people in non-*pitta* climates – just as *Hatha-Yoga* also aimed its yoga at the *pitta* and *rajasic Gurkha* warriors, not for the average person of northern India outside this constitution, aggressive *kshatriya* nature, or climate. They were also required to fight in the hot, dry desert regions in *Sindh* to the

Middle-East, which is why high intake of dairy, raw foods etc. worked well for them alone.

This of course doesn't mean we give meats for all diseases! It simply means adopting the foods one is accustomed to and tailoring such as per their disease, which sometimes means reducing or complete cutting out these or placing one on a bland diet at times.

This contradicts the view of New-Age Ayurveda which argues (on moral grounds) that one and all must adopt the Indian vegetarian diets for health and in diseased cases! It is in fact a clear violation of Ayurvedic principles and tenets as per the classics and would appear to cause more difficulty long-term, especially considering the strange diets of today such as veganism that don't even agree with ancient lacto-vegetarian models!

In continuing this discussion, *Charaka Samhita* (*Chikitsasthana,* XXX.320) states that a physician that doesn't take these local suitable considerations relative to *desha* (location, geographical suitability etc.), age, strength of the patient and their body into account and simply prescribes therapies alone is a failure.

He continues (ibid, 321 – 325) giving examples of, just as how the diets of Chinese, Europeans etc. doesn't affect them, though sometimes contrary to disease, so sometimes like qualities of the *doshas* can alleviate them, as pitta deep within the tissues can be brought out by heat as in poultices or hot application and that excreta from a fly, though causing vomiting sensations, can also cure it (things which are normally contrary, but in certain cases help the disorder)!

These are perhaps some of the more important aspects relative to use of meats in Ayurveda we need to take note of, relative to historical and true traditional Ayurveda accounts.

It hence also calls into question the reasoning for adopting such dietary regimes as being so-called *sattvic* (pure) for such modern 'American Ayurveda' protagonists and their brethren, when they ignore the Ayurvedic guidelines in which what is *sattvic* or pure for one person, is not suitable for the constitution of another - and may even cause health-issues (meats for example can be heavy and *tamasic*, but *vata* being light, requires such heavier substances to calm its *rajasic* and ethereal *sattvic* nature; heavy spices are *rajasic* but required to get *kapha*'s sluggish nature moving).

Here, the New-Age and pseudo-Yoga diets can quite dangerous when they ignore local aspects of *desha satmya* or local suitability and customisation.

VII: Ayurveda and Insanity: A Fresh Look at the Classics from a Traditional Viewpoint

Background:

Ayurvedic Psychology has greatly been underestimated in the West, as also distorted by the New-Age Ayurveda which has superimposed its own biases
and misinterpretations upon the system, rather than examine the traditional aspects as seen in the great science itself.

Movements such as the Arya Samaj and its founder, *Maharishi Dayananda Saraswati* often have stressed the need to go back to the original texts and sources of tradition to ascertain the truth in various Hindu sciences, which have been distorted over time. The approach here also follows this line.
As an example, in India, various systems have been developed by lesser-classes, often Buddhist monks in southern India who did not have access to the sacred texts of the Brahmins and were not allowed to study the classical texts in detail and hence developed their own pseudo-systems, which later influenced the mainstream of Hindu society and sciences. An example of this are the *Marmas* or vital energies in Ayurveda.
Marmas are vital spots that require *varma* (armour) or protection. *Sushruta Samhita* (*Sharirasthana*, VI, 41-43) states marmas should not be damaged in any way, which also means no use of acupressure nor acupuncture on them traditionally, as these cause damage and aggravate the *doshas*, which includes cutting, hitting, fire even near the Marma causes issues (*Su. Sam. Sharirasthana*, 35 & 41).

The commentator on the *Sushruta Samhita*, *Dalhana* himself states the definition of Marma is "*Marayanti iti marmani*", which means that a Marma is one which causes death (if damaged).

In his chapter on *Siras* or veins and venesection, *Sushruta* also states that one should avoid all areas where there are *Marmas* for this procedure also. This again alludes to the prohibition of acupressure and acupuncture at the *Marma* sites and shows they are to be avoided and not touched, except for healing purposes (when wounded due to battle, accidents etc.).

Marmas were hence used in battle for the purposes of maiming others and causing various injuries to organs they relate to and should be healed alone, not pushed, prodded or manipulated, which although can produce short-term effects, long-term, would aggravate the *doshas* and cause injuries to organs, as per the Samhitas. They hence formed a part of the science of *Dhanurveda* or Indian Martial Arts, which was taken to China by Buddhist monks around the 5th Century AD, along with Ayurveda, the science to heal them when they were impaired to avoid damage to the vital organs they corresponded to.

Originally, Marmas had their respective oils, pastes and formulas for healing them, reducing swelling (*sophahara*), healing wounds and pains (*vrana-ropana, shulahara*) etc. (*Rig Veda*, X.97.1). Originally, *Marmabhyanga* or *Marma-Massage* included therapies where *Tailas* or oils were used in the reduction of accumulation of *doshas* at the site of the *Marmas*; coconut-based oils and soothing pastes where *Pitta* and bleeding were involved, drying herbs and pastes where *Kapha* was involved with swelling and application of heat-boluses etc. to reduce swelling as also *Tailas* or oils for *Vata* where there was dryness and cracking at *Marma* sites to counter this - which also involves processes such as *Shirodhara* for the head-marmas (region of *Pranavayu*), when *Vata* invaded the head *Marmas* and so on.

So likewise, forms of Cancer, which are numerous in Ayurvedic texts have also been limited in the West to the three *doshas* - viz. *Vata* (ether and air), *Pitta* (fire and water) and *Kapha* (water and earth) alone. Treatment has become more spiritual and herbal and adopted an anti-surgical approach, which contradicts all of the classical Ayurvedic texts, which note of 13 major types of tumours or cancers including *doshic* forms. Within these exist several sub-categories - for example, *Twak-Arbuda* or skin-cancer falls under the *rakta* or blood and *pitta* (bile) categories, as *rakta* or blood itself is related to *Pitta* and causes issues on the skin. The blood hence had to be purified for such issues. Then there are cancers as per various locations of the body. There are also forms of *granthis* or tumours such as *Gulma* or abdominal tumours, dealt with at length in the Ayurvedic texts.

There are for example other forms detailed in the Ayurvedic classics such as *oshta-arbuda* (lip-cancer), having forms as *mamsarboda, jalarbuda, medorbuda* and *arbuda, Talu-arbuda* or cancer of the palate, *Galarbuda* or cancer of the throat, *Mukharbuda* or cancer of the mouth (cavity), *Karna-arbuda* (cancer of the ears), *Nasa-arbuda* (cancer of the nose), *Netrarbuda* (cancer of the eye), *Kapala-arbuda* (cancer of the skull) etc. and their treatment by *shastrakarma* (surgical intervention) by cutting out the tumours and cauterising the area, or by cauterisation and alkalis alone, depending on their size and stage of advacement. Herbal therapies were given as supplements to these therapies, not as cures, much like modern medicine with requires surgery and use of radiation therapy (the updated form of cauterisation).

So likewise, Ayurvedic Psychology has been limited to a science of possession by wicked entities, gods, demons and ghosts in the New Age Ayurveda, which sees such disorders as Schizophrenia as simply psychic-possession, without actually even noting the philosophy behind these, or that Ayurveda considers various forms of insanity - arising from the *doshas* to external factors such as poisons, such as we will discuss here in greater detail.

First of all however, we have to understand the background of Psychological profiling in Ayurveda and also a deeper understanding of what is meant by the so-called entities or organisms than produce the *bhuta* or *graha* - the supernatural types of insanity in Ayurveda, from a traditional point of view.

Ayurvedic Psychological Types and Insanity:

The classical Ayurvedic texts or *Samhitas* tell us that there are various varieties of people according to their psyche - from a *Brahma* (supreme) to a *Vanaspatya* (tree) type, according to mentality or psychic constitution (*Manasic Prakriti*).

These types are elaborated below:

1.Sattvic types:

Brahma:

A Brahma-type person represents the highest type, that of Brahma or the Supreme. Such a person will exhibit extraordinary divine traits (*para-sattvic*). Such people are said to be engaged in the study of the religious texts (*Vedas*) and performing rituals such as the fire-sacrifices regularly. Such types are seen only in *avatars*, the divine incarnations of the Supreme on earth or in human form and is hence seldom seen. The *Prajapatis*, the progenitors of mankind, as also *Manu* the first man are in this category.

Rishi:

A Rishi type is like a Brahma-type and represents the *Mahasattvas* or the quality of Great sattvas or purity. Like the Brahma-type, such types are rare and seen only in a few Yogis of modern India even. Such people will be engaged in the *yamas* and *niyamas* of Yoga and study of the texts, celibacy, meditation, sacrifices and have wisdom of the higher cosmic principles. The ancient *Yoga-Rishis* such as *Patanjali, Vishwamitra* and *Sri Krishna* are in this category.

Indra:

An Indra-type person is one who is like *Mahendra*, the lord of the demigods and as such is commanding, full of courage and knowledge and protects others. The ideal man and King of ancient India, *Sri Rama* was an Indra-type personality. This represents the stage of worldly or ordinary *sattvas* of man as the ideal role-model for others.

Yama:

A Yama-type represents the nature of the god of death. Such a person performs actions with determination and at the appropriate times and is fearless, without passion or delusions. Such a type requires adherence to the Divine Laws however. Such a person represents the stage of *Sattvas mixed with rajas* or the quality of goodness, but with some passion or action or pride (*rajas*) inherit in their nature, required in order for them to uphold the divine law and justice.

Varuna:

A Varuna-type is similar to a Yama-type, but is more purely *rajasic* level under the *sattvic* umbrella and represents the level of the chief of the lesser-gods. Such a person is said to be well-spoken and desires cold and has brown body, hair and eyes, denoting valour.

Kubera:

A Kubera type is one who is the mid-road human, the person of a sattvic disposition but with the quality of *rajas mixed with tamas* under this. Such people are charitable and are wealthy (due to past *rajasic samskaras*) and often have many children. They are able to withstand difficulties quite well.

Gandharva:

The Gandharva is the last sub-type of the *sattvic* types and represents its *tamasic* stage, the lowest of the sattvic types. Such a person is desirous of perfumes, garlands, fine things in life and also music, dance and fine foods. They may indeed be talented artists and musicians. Yet, as they lowest state of *sattvic* types, they are just above the level of ordinary *rajas* in people, seen by their more materialistic pursuits.

2. Rajasic types:

Asura:

The Asura type is the *Maha-sattvic* or greater or better *rajasic* type of person, owing to some sattvas. Such people are very monumental and desire and have much wealth, courage but also traits of anger, and jealously and can be gluttons. Such a temperament is a materialistic businessperson who is overweight and has wealth and power in society and seeks to keep it that way! Asuras can be very devotional to the Gods, which makes them a greater *sattvic* type under *rajasic.*

Rakshasa:

A Rakshasa type is a more worldly *Sattvic-based* or higher type under the *rajasic* personalities below the *Asura.* Such a person is like an Asura type but of a lower kind and capable of understanding things by themselves but more terrifying and jealous in nature that often has a large ego and often transgresses the social norm or laws. Such people are the typical white-collar criminals and such of society who take pride in ripping off the system or the tax-man and feel no remorse in doing so!

Pishacha:

The Pishacha type person is the sattvic-*rajasic* type that is *rajas mixed with sattvas* or better qualities but still mixed with passion and aggression. Such a person scavenges foods which have been left behind are not shy and are very lustful. Such people we can see with criminals in society or the homeless who move from place to place and scrounges for food off the streets and by begging.

Sarpa:

A Sarpa, the lowest purely *rajasic* type of a more *rajasic* nature and such as type is of the nature of a serpent. Such people are fickle-minded, fast in nature, always changing place or abode, angry and aggressive, deceptive and likes recreational pastimes. We see such people as people who have undergone severe mental trauma or drug abuse in life, but seek to blame others for their predicament. They seldom seek help and when they do, they are seldom successful due to the waves of previous *rajasic samskaras* from the past mixed with the *rajasic samskaras* in this life that they have picked up and added to their state. They can be intelligent however!

Preta:

A Preta type is a purely *tamasic-rajasic* or mixed kind of the *rajasic* category of people, like a ghost. Such a type is lazy, possessive, jealous, sensuous and likes to hoard things and not give anything to others. Such types are always plagued by anxiety and distress. Such types are those who hard that much that they turn their homes or environments into living garbage tips and never seek to remove their clutter.

Shakuna:

A Shakuna is a bird-type personality and we can see this as an expression of the lowest *tamasic* level of the *rajasic* types. Such a type is mobile like a bird and does not stay in one play long and always distressed and always impatient and always consuming foods. It is placed just above the purely *tamasic* types owing to it being a bird - an animal.

3. Tamasic types:

Pashava:

The Pashava or beastly type is one who acts like an animal and represents the *sattvic* or higher stage under the greater *tamasic* level. Such people always think negative thoughts, are slow in whatever they do, has many dreams and is lustful as well as denying their own issues and problems. Such people are very difficult to be helped and are sloths.

Matsya:

The Matsya is the fish-personality, representing *rajas* under the *tamasic* level. Like a fish, such people are unsteady, dull in intellect or ignorant people, always fearing something, always fighting with people and desire water and dense objects. Such people are the ignorant followers of blind faiths or religions and cults that do whatever others say without question.

Vanaspatya:

The final type is the Vanaspatya or tree-type. This type of personality is the lowest, the *tamasic* type under the *tamasic* umbrella. Such people are dead and inert in emotions and feelings like a tree. They like only to eat and will not go out or travel and have no wealth and never speak the truth. Such people are vegetables of society who would rather sit and complain about everything and do nothing. Such types are those who also are reborn into lesser animal forms in their next lives if they do not change their behaviours as they attract or create more negative *samskaras* and *vasanas* or impressions in their minds.

Charaka Samhita (Nidanasthana, VII.5) states that *unmada* (insanity) is seen due to a perversion of the mind, intellect, consciousness, knowledge, memory, desire and behavioral patterns. Any of these above types hence also represents a shift or change in attitude according to their mental constitution in the classical texts and hence the various traits that are seen in these various types.

The main causes of insanity are due to aggravations on the biological constitutions or *doshas* in the body, such as *Vata* (ether and air - breath or movement), *Pitta* (fire and water - bile and blood) and *Kapha* (water and earth - lubrication and phlegm).

Basic types of insanity in the texts are *Vataja* (Vata-type), *Pittaja* (Pitta-type), *Kaphaja* (Kapha-type), *Sannipata* (all three *doshas* together) and *Agantuja* (external factors such as divorce, shock, grief and also poisons or toxins etc.). These types are distinguished from the *bhuta* types that we will also discuss, also known as *graha* or seizures.

Thus according to afflictions also, there are also *Deva, Pishacha, Yaksha, Rakshasa* etc. types of *graha* or seizures upon the mind, which are caused as a result of ridiculing or imitating such beings or classes of men. *Sarngadhara Samhita (I.7.37-39)* describes 20 types of possession-caused insanity: *Deva, Danava, Gandharva, Kinnara, Yaksha, Pitr, Guhyaka, Preta,* by *Vriddhas, Siddhas, Bhutas, Pishachas, Jala-Devatas, Nagas, Brahmarakshasas, Rakshasas, Kushmandas, Vetalas,* by *Krityonmada* (caused by actions such as magic etc.) and by the curse of the Guru.

On this note, imitation here also resonates with modern New-Age practices such as Reiki and Pranic Healing etc., where the person imitates the *Deva* or God with healing powers. According to Ayurveda, by way of karmic effects (cause and effect as a result of this), one can come down with insanity. Likewise, practices such as Channeling are also inferred here, as they could bring about *possession* according to Ayurveda, of these various types of entities (airborne bacteria) as a result of creating a *tamasic* or negative environment (excess *prana / vata* or air, causing depletion in *ojas* or vitality in the body and the bodily tissues, thus allowing such bacteria or viruses to impair the person and their psyche easier). Channeling and Pranic Healing as they are today actually find no mention in Hindu texts - *Pranic Healing* simply was confined to healing via *Pranayama* or breathing techniques with their psycho-physical effects and eradication of disease by breathing out toxins in the body and oxygenating the blood and brain. It was a rational system.

Affliction of these types of 'entities' however also relates to classes of physical human people or tribes as well.

Pishachas generally denoted the Dardic people of the Himalaya such as the Dards and Kalash, who are nomadic tribes. *Yakshas* and *Rakshasas* also denote the people of Sri Lanka in earlier times and the *Devas* were the people of northern India into the Himalayas. *Kinnaras* and *Gandharvas* were in the performing arts, *Nagas* were the people of eastern-India and into south-east Asia (with their dragons and serpents) and so on. *Nagas* being serpents also relates to insanity being caused by being bitten by a snake or terrorised by them as well. Apparitions and hallucinations come into effect here with relation to these various classes of "entities" as well.

Yet, these also denote subtle viruses etc. as well, but causes of insanity arising due to the physical element (harassing or ridiculing tribes) we can infer, was hence due to physical afflictions these people produced upon them as a consequence of direct harassment (threatening their families, robbing them, public humiliation etc.) or as a consequence of supernatural factors, such as the law of *karana* (cause) and *karya* (effect), known as *karma*. A guilty conscience is hence also a possible causative factor here also, if we interpret in this broad manner, the texts appear to state.

It also appears then, as a culture, that by breeding new viruses and bacteria, we are actually getting back our own negative karma. Maharishi Dayananda Saraswati on this stated that we should all daily perform the *Agni Hotra* or fire-offerings which help purify the air, prevent bacteria and help the atmosphere and hence Mother Earth. By neglecting this and creating a culture of pollution and arrogance, it appears that the negative bacteria are the negative side as a karmic result of neglecting these and also the native people of the Earth also (for example driving away native tribes to develop their land into housing complexes etc. for the wealthy, converting Brahmins to Christianity and Islam etc., which brings about negative karmic reactions for a whole nation and individually, which appears to come in the form of viruses, insanity and such - which do plague our society now, more than ever!).

We shall describe what these various types actually denote later on.

Subtly (karmically), these classifications are known to be linked to the cycles of Astrology as the Rishis understood affliction could occur at certain times, just as the Moon influences the tides. We can classify these as being caused by (a) viruses or bacteria causing insanity and (b) various classes of insanity outside the *doshic* forms that the *Samhitas* list, as *Bhutonmada* or insanity as a result of spirits - or rather, the elements (meaning external factors due to environment, dust, parasites, bacteria, fear, traumas, accidents, storms or viruses etc.). *Bhuta* here means the *Panchamahabhutas* or caused by the physical world, which according to *Samkhya* (cosmological) philosophy, is a creation of the five great elements. The terms as *rakshasa* etc. here are hence subdivisions of such that afflict the mind.

Hinduism understands atomism through its *Vaisheshika* philosophy also, which comprehends subatomic particles (*paramanus*) as the building blocks of all creation. I hence understand the concept of subtle parasites or micro-organisms existing as well, as a consequence of this philosophy.

On this, Charaka (*Charaka Samhita, Sutrasthana, XI.45*) clarifies that *Bhuta*-caused means the elements - viz. *vishavayu* (poisoned air), *agni* (fire and heat) etc.and *Manasa* (mentally-caused) are due to emotional upsets etc. as unfulfilled desires. The 20 types mentioned in *Sarngadhara Samhita* hence have their origins here. *Krityonmada*, caused by magic etc. would be due to trying to perform actions to gain wealth, supernatural powers etc. and due to a failure of such, one falls into insanity (as in cases of anxiety-depression etc.). Curse of a Guru can be described as (a) karmic, but also as a result of one's Guru or teacher chastising them or (b) taking away titles and positions of the disciple, causing grief and hence mental agony causing depression -

similar to what we have noted relative to microorganisms and tribes of people by their *karmic* effects or physical insults causing mania (logically speaking - we will discuss karma further on).

Sushruta (*Sushruta Samhita, Uttarasthana,* LX.5) states that these *grahas* (bhutas) possess a person who is wounded or not, unclean in habits (inferring bacteria) etc. which also reveals these as airborne bacteria and subject to external toxins, viruses and so forth. He also states (*Uttarasthana,* LX.37), that is they do no go away by chanting of mantras etc. (sound-effects and spiritual therapies for the mind or Psycho-therapy), then they should be treated with medical drugs.

Bhava Prakasha (*Madhya Khanda,* 52.49) on contagious skin diseases also lists fevers, ulcers and specifically *Bhutonmada* (insanity caused by *bhutas* or supernatural forces / elements, as noted here) to be passed on through sexual intercourse, breath (i.e airborne bacteria or viruses specifically – Ayurvedic texts list *krimi* as parasites directly) from clothes, sharing foods etc. of infected people. Hence, this also confirms again these are bacteria and viruses.
   We can hence also see these as productions of various toxins in the environment that cause chemical imbalances in the mind. Another example of a toxic involvement of the senses is the Television and News media and also Social-media, through which we must also develop an attitude of Pratyahara and sensory withdrawal from also, as such impressions can also create disturbances in our psyche and can create bad dreams, as the great author *Vagbhata* itself states:

*"Bad dreams are the result of blocks in the manovahasrotas (mind carrying channels), due to toxins in the body." -**Ashtanga Hridaya, Sharirasthana**,*VI.59-60

Understanding this, the Vedic people developed methods such as the *Agni-Hotra* or *Homa* with various *yajnas* which helped by offering substances into the fire and (a) bringing about a subtle change in climate at the causal level as well as (b) purifying the atmosphere and physical surroundings by offering special herbs and herbal combinations that were anti-bacterial in nature to help kill off microorganisms, thus preventing viruses, bacteria and hence diseases causing both psychological and also somatic diseases.

We often misunderstand such ancient sciences, although the ancient *Vedas* of India, in the original *Sanskrit,* as well as other text speak volumes of them. The classical Ayurvedic texts also speak about other forms of *krimi* (microbial organisms). *Madhava Nidana* and other texts speak volumes of them, stating they are very small to even invisible ad enter into the blood-system affecting the person (*Madhana Nidana* VII.11-12). Some forms of heart diseases (bacterial endocarditis) and headaches in Ayurveda are also caused by these microorganisms, revealing the ancient advanced nature and complexity of the science.

That Ayurveda has a special and extensive "special" branch of microbiology (*bhutas, grahas* – those arising from the elements and natural environment and "seize" the individual's body through infection) that is solely attached to the science of Psychology, is in itself, evidence of the advanced and scientific nature of the ancient Ayurvedic physicians, who understood that not merely *doshic* forces were behind psychological disorders and unrest alone.

Ayurveda and Yoga hence recognise several states of the mind and several causative factors for this, as noted by these types and also the Psychic Types, such as *Brahma, Indra* etc types also. Other forms of Indian philosophy describe several other types, as also by *lokas* (spheres of realms of consciousness), such as represented by the 14 major *chakras* in Hinduism, which correspond to these numerous states of being or psychology. In many Yoga systems, there are actually 21 chakras, each with their own three levels of consciousness according to *sattvas, rajas* and *tamas*, thus giving a total of 63 broad states of consciousness.

Many schools of *Shaivite Hinduism* and Yoga also have the view that there are also seven higher planes (paracausal) of consciousness beyond *Brahmaloka* (the highest plane) or the *Sahasrarachakra* (crown chakra) which many systems see as being the "liberated" state of the Soul also. The great Yogi *Gorakshanatha* refers to the state of *Paramashunya* or the Transcendental Void beyond the 21 Chakras itself for example (including the seven *Parasiva Chakras of Saiva Siddhanta* above the *Sahasradala* or thousand-petalled lotus / Crown chakra). This gives us several more states of consciousness regarding the mind.

These three states Yoga and Ayurveda recognise under which various levels of the mind can be influenced or operate - viz. *sattvas* (purity, clarity and truth), *rajas* (passion, agitation or aggravation) and *tamas* (delusion, darkness and ignorance) thus play a major factor in understanding Psychology from the Indian point of view traditionally. Sub-divisions also exist, such as a mixture of *sattvas* (purity) and *rajas* (passion), mixtures of *rajas* (passion) and *tamas* (ignorance) etc. giving us essentially five broader states (*sattvas, sattvas-rajas, rajas, rajas-tamas* and *tamas*).

Jainism recognises six *leshyas* viz. *shukla* (white), *padma* (yellow), *tejo* (red), *kapot* (grey), *neela* (blue) and *kala* (black) according to these, which correspond to these various mental states.

These three states Yoga and Ayurveda recognise under which various levels of the mind can be influenced or operate - viz. *sattvas* (purity, clarity and truth), *rajas* (passion, agitation or aggravation) and *tamas* (delusion, darkness and ignorance) thus play a major factor in understanding Psychology from the Indian point of view traditionally.

The *Rig Veda*, the oldest texts of the Hindus alludes to 99 states of the mind (refer to my book, 'Vaidik Para-Yoga Vijnana'), or rather, levels of consciousness one can become entrapped in.

Buddhist Psychology also mentions various factors, such as in *Abhidhammatt-sangaha* - 52 mental factors are noted by them, including 14 unwholesome factors or the mind. Such should be studied also, with regards to these on deeper levels, as they contain older teachings of the Samkhya and Yoga schools that were lost.

This is also reflected in the treatment of Psychological disorders, as mentioned in the Ayurvedic text, Ashtanga Hridayam and here we also reflect relative to techniques as *Pranayama* for purifying the mind and body and the state of the bodily tissues, relative to a sound mind:

"The pure state of the indriyas (sensory organs), objects, the discerning power of intellect and reason (buddhi), soul and mind, as well as the normal-funtioning state of the [seven] bodily tissues (dhatus) are signs of an individual that has been freed in psychological unrest" - **Ashtanga Hridayam, Uttara Sthana, VI.60**

The *buddhi* or intellect itself is hence deranged by delusion and also colourings of *rajas* and *tamas* in the mind, which can be due to various parasites and micro-organisms or viruses that can also afflict them.

The Rig Veda also notes on various parasites and mental disorders, related to them, if we translate the terms correctly, as I have noted in the following verse:

"The Deva expels all the rakshasas and yatudhanas, with all those offensive defects (prati-dosham, Vikriti) and hatred." **Rig Veda. I.35.10**

Rakshasas are those who injure, destroy etc. *Yatudhanas* are another class of *rakshasas*. *Prati-dosham* can also mean the "offensive *dosha*", or the vitiated *dosha* (*vikara*), depending on how we translate the term.

Dosha itself is a synonym for *roga* (disease), *vikara* (deviation from nature nature) etc. which is connected to the term *dushya*, meaning a defect vitiation etc.
Here, the hymn relates to these causing disease and driving them off. *Surya* (Sun) as the *Deva* is the Light or "Shining One" that drives them off, relating the Light against Darkness (*Tamas*), or the force of heat against disease, parasites and bacteria (*krimi*), of which *rakshasa* and *yatudhana* are Vedic synonyms. They also mean bacteria, infections, viruses and such also. It also refers to the fire of discrimination (*vivekagni*) that negates *avidya* or ignorance in the mind, which is also a causative factor of insanity, due to the improper association of the mind and hence creating delusions or even hallucinations (such as the false belief one has seen a ghost, god, demon or is possessed by them) and such by mistaking on object for another, as a snake for a rope (*Shankaracharya, Vivekachudamani*, 138).

The first part of the above Rig-Vedic hymn lauds *Savitar* or the Sun as "*Hiranya-hasta*" or "Golden handed", which on this note does not mean the God himself, but relates to *Haridra* (Haldi) or Turmeric, which is well-known to have famous anti-bacterial properties, when used internally (as a *rakta-shodhaka dravya* - blood-purifying agent) and also externally (as a *vrana-shodhaka* - wound-healing agent). In the same verse, Savitar is lauded as the "*Asura*", which comes from *asu* (breath) and *ra* (ruling force) or "ruling-life breath", meaning *Asura* is another term for *Prana*. And Prana also means *Vata* here. Thus, the *Hiranya-hasta* (Haridra) connected to *Asura* (Prana) here shows that it increases *Prana* or *Vata*, also relating to the symbolic wisdom of the Rig Veda stating Haridra or Turmeric is a Vata-increasing herb that here drives away infection, parasites and such.
As noted, *Rakshasa, Yakshasa, Yatudhana, Pishacha, Gandharva* etc. are all synonyms for *Krimi* or Viruses, Bacteria, Parasites or Disease (*Roga*) in the Vedic texts, such as the Atharva Veda, where they can be understood in their proper context in the science of

microbiology, in these symbolic lights. Vata-Dosha is also the main cause of severe psychological disorders or derangement in the Ayurvedic classics also. In the context of viruses and bacteria, the Ayurvedic classics, such as *Sushruta Samhita* also have charms and special fumigation to help protect against them - the term used again is *rakshasa*,

Modern science also recognises factors such as herpes and other viruses as also causative factors of Schizophrenia. The Hindu *Atharvaveda*, from which Ayurveda is said to have arisen also has many hymns extolling various viruses, bacteria and other micro-organisms and their cure as well. Issues as depression etc. are also seen to be caused by microorganisms as per modern findings [2]
Brahmarakshasa type psychic disorder is one of the most severe forms of insanity in the Ayurvedic texts and is said to be characterised by one hating priests, religious texts, physicians etc. (inferring here, they do not adhere to the laws of the land or moral ethics and codes) and also injure themselves (*Charaka, Chikitsasthana*, IX.20) and comes on during a full-moon, which has been associated with lunacy (hence the term) - mainly due to it's factor to historically affect sleep patterns. The ancients however did believe that the lunar cycles did produce various effects upon the psyche, which modern science is yet to research more - and of which are noted in the Ayurvedic texts as being factors also causing insanity. Some noted Psychiatrists such as Ian Stevenson **(1)** are also well-known to have documented accounts of reincarnation scientifically. Carl Jung **(2)** the noted Psychologist was also open regarding the effects of Astrology and the birth-chart as is well-known.

As noted however, Ayurvedic classics that the cause of these effects or disorders, is karmic and due to negative karmic actions in the past (*Charaka Samhita, Nidanasthana, VII.10, VII.19-20*). Likewise, while Ayurveda recognises that *atmaja* (genetic) disorders derives from the ovum or sperm or mother or father, the primal or *karana* (causal) form of this is also karmic, and causes afflictions as a result in the embryo, as also to the psyche (below taken from PV Sharma translation, Chaukhambha Orientalia, Varanasi, reprinted edition, 2011):

"All foetuses have four elements (all except ether – viz. wind, fire, water and earth) which are fourfold also as maternal, paternal, nutritional and self-borne. Because of them the dominant factors arise from past-life deeds of the parents and resemble the physical appearance. Likewise the mental state is also determined by the past lives or species."
-Charaka Samhita, Shaririasthana, II.23-27,

"According to past karmas (actions), form arises from form and mind from mind. Whatever difference is seen in the physique and psyche is caused by rajas (passion) and tamas (darkness, ignorance) as well as the past karmas."
-Charaka Samhita, Sharirasthana, II.36

Charaka Samhita (*Vimanasthana, VIII.95*) also confirms that by the constitution of the sperm and ovum, food and behaviour of the Mother and of the products of the five

---

[2] Modern research shows that depression could be caused by bacteria. Source:
http://www.dailymail.co.uk/health/article-2850645/Could-depression-INFECTIOUS-DISEASE-Condition-caused-parasites-bacteria-virus-prevented-jab-expert-claims.html

elements, the *dosha* or the *Prakriti*, the biological constitutional nature of the individual becomes manifest as such – either *Vata, Pitta, Kapha* or a combination thereof.

Diseases (*Vikriti*) however are another issue and come out as a result of past karmas or seeds and actions that one does and affects us also:

"Deeds in previous lives are known as 'Daiva' (divine) and those from the present life as 'Paurusha' (pertaining to man). These in an unbalanced manner cause diseases, when in balance they avoid them." **-Charaka Samhita, Sharirasthana, II.44 (PV Sharma Translation)**

Gandharva type is characterised as if one is "possessed" by a musician and has similar traits. Karmically, the cause here is said to be ridiculing musicians or dancers in a former life and hence such *vasanas* or mental impressions are lodged in the subtle mind-stuff or consciousness (*chitta*) and come out in the future life as a psychic derangement. Thus, some are not produced by bacteria as such, but as a result of past-life actions and subtle mental impressions or *stains* if we like, that come out in the next life as traits suddenly. *Gandharva* type is said to come out on the twelfth and fourteenth days of the lunar fortnight, which accounts again for the subtle-effects of the external world or effects of the lunar cycles, as also according to one's own karma or destiny as per his past-life actions. The science behind such psychic derangement in the classical texts then, is quite specific and goes beyond the spheres known to modern psychologists.

However, the commentator on *Charaka Samhita*, Chakrapani (commentating on *Sutrasthana, I.54*) also states that *prajaparadha* or perversion of the intellect causes one to commit bad deeds (karmas). Taking of impure foods, insulting teachers and learned people (Brahmins), mental shock, fear and irregular or forced bodily movements cause insanity. This causes the bodily biological humours to become aggravated and dulls the truth-perception or reality of the person (*sattvas*) in the heart (of the mind), enter the mental-channels and derange the mind of the person (*Charaka, Chikitsasthana, IX.4-5*). This also means taking incompatible foods such as milk with seafoods, artificial poisons or emotions such as anger (*krodha*), which can damage the mind, according to *Chakrapani*, the commentator on Charaka Samhita.
As a result of this, Ayurveda employs various exotic methods of imparting *sattvas* or purity to the mind, by way of various devotional practices such as *poojas* (devotional offerings), *seva* (selfless service or volunteer work), *dhana* (charity), *havanas* (fire-offerings), which cultivate detachment, bring in the idea of *sattvas* (purity) and *dharma* (righteousness) to the person by such psychotherapy techniques.
The *Havana* is also known to destroy airborne bacteria, viruses and also impart nice smells etc. which are pleasing to the psyche, as also by the fire itself, awakens *vivekagni* or discrimination and mental metabolism in people, which is not properly functioning when there is insanity. Various medications and reciting hymns (music therapy) are also noted in the texts, as well as specific herbs and formulas for the mind to help clear the *manovahasrotas* or mental channels of impurities or chemical imbalances and impart proper cognitive functions to the mind.

These rituals also help to reduce the *karana-nidanas* or causal factors that have caused them - the karmic factors as "karmic reduction methods" by accruing *punya karmas* (good karmas) and positive *vasanas* or mental traits as a result and forcing out the *papa-karmas* or bad actions that have caused these (before the genetic and other stages - i.e. why we are fated with such diseases or issues). They hence have no "magical" or "supernatural" effects of their own with relation to Deities and such, but simply work upon altering our karmas or subtle causative factors that have brought thus about, by our own wrong-doings. By imparting *sattvas* or clarity and truth to the mind physically, this acts subtly also on our *chitta* or mind-stuff that stores all past *vasanas* or *samskaras* (karmic mental traits and impressions of past-lives) and transforms them, as it were, thus altering the (physical) outcome of the disease as a result (rectifying the root-cause of these).

Charaka (*Charaka Samhita, Sutrasthana, XI.46, 54*) states of these therapies, that they are there to keep the mind freed of unwholesome objects (or from performing bad actions, further complicating the disease) and hence their employment in treatment (*mano-nigraha* - attempts to subdue the mind), which constitutes *Sattvavajaya* or psychological therapies - of which *Daivavyapashraya*, the "divine therapies" or spiritual therapies hence form an integral part of and are done along with *Yuktivyapashraya*, that is, rational therapies as diet, herbs and formulas for the mind. Shock-therapies were also given in various cases according to the specific mental derangement also. Charaka thus states that opposite therapies according to the mental disorder (*Sutrasthana, XI.46*) should be adopted, which proves such "spiritual therapies" were mental distractions and psychological tools for also providing detachment of the mind, mental disorder etc. Charaka (*Chikitsasthana, IX.96*) also states that insanity can be avoided if one abstains from eating meats and wines or impure diets etc. and hence are seen as causative factors (*nidanas*) of various kinds of insanity. Various meats and also alcohol are given various factors or qualities (*gunas*) in Ayurveda, according to their chemical reactions upon the mind, which are described as aggravating *rajas* and *tamas* in the mental channels, blurring our perceptions. As such, they are to be avoided in such conditions. Various *dosha*-aggravating factors are also listed in the classical texts according to their variations of disorder as well.

We hence see that there is a great depth of Psychology and causative factors behind mental derangement in the Ayurvedic texts with a rational basis. Whereas western medicine stops short of genetic factors, Ayurveda questions how these genetic factors affect the individual directly themselves, which is a consequence of past-life karmas causing such specific afflictions to the mind, that have to be rectified by spiritual methods or *Sattvavajaya*, that is, imparting purity and clarity to the mind through various psychological tools, *vairagya* (detachment) that they help cultivate (as an attitude of 'giving' rather than 'clinging' or attachment to them).

As such, Yoga is one of the tools here that also helps take the mind away from the attachment of one's past deeds or *karmas* and thus helps in restoring the body and mind back to health:

"Happiness and misery are due to contact with the Self (Atman), mind and senses, but when the mind is steadily concentrated on the Self, both cease to exist, due to non-initiation and a supernatural power comes forth from the person. This state is known as Yoga by the seers" -**Charaka Samhita, Sharirasthana, I.137 (PV Sharma translation)**

Thus, while modern American Ayurveda has sought to turn Ayurvedic Psychology into some mumbo-jumbo or help promote it as a pseudo-science in the West, the Vedic tradition represents a highly sophisticated model with further truths beyond what is currently known to western Psychology and also various techniques that were seen as simply tools in aiding the mind to restore it back to health, rather than magical powers of Divinities etc.

Deeper Meaning of Afflictions by Devas and Rishis:

We have noted the various afflictions by forms of *possession* and their meaning various as airborne parasites and also karmic conditions arising out of impurities in the mind and use of meat and wine etc. However, as per the Deva and Rishi types, there are also other specific considerations, relative to their symbolism. As noted, there are several levels to these, but here we also express yet another level of how they can cause psychic disturbances, according to their Vedic interpretations.

Some examples are already seen in the *Upanishads*, such as the *Brihadaranyaka Upanishad* (II.2.4) which correlates the so-called *Rishis* or Seers as the two ears(*Gotama* and *Bharadvaja*); the two eyes (*Vishwamitra* and *Jamadagni*); the two nostrils (*Vasishtha* and *Kashyapa*) and *Rishi Atri* is the tongue. As such, these respective "*Rishis*" denote the various organs connected to the *Nadis* or subtle currents in Yoga also. The term *Ganga* (Ganges) is often translated as it, but also refers to a *Nadi* or subtle current in Yoga, plus means standing or being near land (*Nighantu, 1.1*).

It is also well-known that of the 33 *Devas* or deities in the texts, that as per *Brihadaranyaka Upanishad.* The 8 *Vasu* deities represent heaven / light (*dyaus*), atmosphere (*antariksha*), wind (*vayu*), fire (*agni*), earth (*prithivi*) as also the sun (*surya*), the moon (*chandrama*) and stars (*nakshatras).* In Vedic Astrology, the *nakshatra* or lunar mansion one is born under is also said to give an insight into their basic psychology, which also represents a deeper level beyond the physical state, that needs to be examined by modern science. However, relative to the Vasus basically here meaning the elements and their impact upon the individuals psyche by their environment and reflection (of the sun, moon, stars, phobias etc.). The 12 *Adityas* are the months of the year (accounting for climatic changes and impacts on the psyche by *dosha*-aggravation as per the seasons). The 11 *Rudras* are the various 10 *Pranas* or breaths in man, which also have their various states and when impaired, cause diseases of both physical and psychic natures also in Yoga and Ayurvedic sciences (the 11th is the *Self* or soul). The remaining two are *Indra*, representing lightening (or physical phenomenon as lightening and storms producing fears, anxieties and psychological issues or insanity in people as a result) and *Prajapati*, representing *Yajna* or sacrifice (inferring that if one gets too close to the fire when performing fire-offerings or done incorrectly - can produce toxic gases or by affects also afflict the mind).

The *Shatapatha Brahmana* (XII.9.1.1-17) also states that the deities represent various organs in the body of man also. *Varuna* the deity represents the lung and breathing, while *Savitri* is the breath. The *Ashwins* are the eyes, nostrils, ears etc., relating to the *nadis* or subtle currents on the left and right side of the body denoting these respectively, whilst the goddess *Saraswati* is the tongue and speech, representing the *Saraswati Nadi* and so on. Even in the Vedas, the deities were hence taken as (i) proper nouns (ii) spiritual terms and (iii) yogic metaphors.

Impairments to these organs and the *Devas* or *Rishis* that rule them for example (meaning the specific regions of the body and their impairments) can hence create psychic disturbances for people as well. Relating to the nostrils for example, *Nasarbuda* or nasal cancer could cause great psychological strain due to the physical impairment of the individual and the stress they underwent as a result of tumours being removed. As we know, Ayurvedic did employ *Rhinoplasty* or plastic surgery for this purpose of repair. *Saraswati* and *Atri Rishi* representing the tongue would also relate to speech impediments such as stuttering which would also be viewed as a psychic affliction in Ayurveda, as also one causing further psychological unrest as a result of this (due to ridicule and low self-esteem etc.).

Sushruta likewise in his *Sushruta Samhita* also correlates the deities with various organs of the body as well (*Sharirasthana*,I.7):
Brahma is *buddhi* (intellect); **Ishvara** is *ahamkara* (ego); **Chandra** (moon) is *manas* (the mind); **Dishadevas** (directional gods) are the *srotras* (ears); **Vayu** (wind) is *twacha* (skin); **Surya** (sun) is *chakshu* (eyes); **Apa** (water deity) is *rasana* (tongue); **Prithivi** (goddess earth) is the *ghrana* (nose); **Agni** (fire god) is *vacha* (speech tongue); **Indra** is *hasta* (hands); **Vishnu** is *pada* (feet); **Mitra** is *payu* (anus) and **Prajapati** is *upastha* (genitals).

The *Pancha Mahabhutas* or five great element that make up the *doshas*, personified as "deities" - viz. ether, wind, fire, water and earth, all have their own correspondences also. Ether relates to sound and the ear; Wind relates to touch and the skin; Fire relates to sight and the eyes; Water relates to taste and the tongue and Earth relates to smell and the nose. Excesses or deficiencies in any of these hence produce afflictions to the mind-body complex.

We have already discussed the *karma* of these and hence here, the deities related to them also relate to the elements and also abusing or polluting the elements in past lives (such as throwing our garbage and polluting the air; throwing toxic substances into the fire and so on).

Impairments to any of these organs according to the *Bhutas* (elements) they relate to hence also denotes the respective *Deva* that causes the psychic affliction also (hence also why Ayurvedic Psychology is known as *Bhutavidya*). On this also, like *Charaka*, *Sushruta* takes this rational approach (*Sutrasthana,* I.25) and states that *manasika* (psychic) disorders are caused by *krodha* (anger), *shoka* (grief), *bhaya* (fear), *harsha* (exhilaration), *vishada* (sadness), *k ama* (lust), *lobha* (greed) etc. and similarly, *Madhava Nidana* (XX.14-15) states insanity is brought on my fright, loss of wealth, death of family members, excessive sexual desire etc. which also further infers these are due to mutations, issues etc. of these various organs constituting the *Deva* class (here *Devas* represent cognition of the organs / senses and elements).

The classics are hence quite logical with regards to various forms of insanity and don't simply ascribe them to supernatural powers, psychic possession etc. simply as has occurred in Western New-Age modifications of the science of Ayurveda. They are viewed as psychic disorders brought on by physical factors, but as a causative result of negative actions (bad karma) from the past. As a result, impairments to bodily organs afflicting the mind, as also other external (mental) factors can also produce insanity falling under the class of *Bhutonmada* or elemental forces or caused by supernatural powers (symbolically only, 'Gods' representing various organs and functioning of the body).

For example, *switra* (leucoderma) would be seen as a *Vayu-type* psychic disorder - meaning one affecting the skin and thereby due to this pigmentation, causing anxiety to the person causing diseases. *Ishvara* type would be due to *ahamkara* or ego and hence creates a kind of narcissism in the person and so on. These *Devas* and *Rishis* as causes of psychic disturbances then have their own sub-classifications that must be understood in their correct context for causing *Unmada* or insanity and here are quite specific, if we look at the classical texts.

They hence shape the mind of the person and produce
various *rajasic* and *tamasic vasanas* or mental impressions as a result, which cause the mind to become unstable, leading to these forms of insanity. No doubt however, that regardless, their initial causes are still a result of negative actions or karmas in the past, which come out as a result in these various diseases. Here, insults to
the *Rishis* and *Devas* could also mean polluting elements or harming the bodily organs of another or insulting another's deformities (especially a Brahmin or teacher - say blind or deaf), which produces subtle karmic patterns or *vasanas* impressions or mental blockages and stains that as a result, produce such disorders of insanity as mentioned above. This is indeed quite a complex science in itself!

In the *Rig Veda*, the antagonist is called *Vritra* or obstruction. He is the father of the God *Indra*. We read from the *Brihadaranyaka Upanishad* that the Father is the Mind (I.V.7) thus also noting this direct affliction. The term *vritra* is also related to *vritti* which are waves or movements of the mind in Yoga, which are to be checked, by controlling the senses (*indriyas*). Indra here is the master of these *indriyas* or senses. We have mentioned before about the role of Yoga and the mind.

By withdrawing our minds and bodies away from such things, we can hence go far in Yoga by cultivating this fire of detachment and withdrawal and therefore help us in restraining the senses overall, by which we can become great Yogis and become free from these *grahas* or seizures/ influences by the Deities and such:

"Restraining speech in the mind and restraining the mind in the intellect; this again restrains in the witness of the intellect and merging with the Supreme Self, attain to the highest peace. The body, the breaths, organs, mind and intellect and others – with whatsoever of these supervening adjuncts of the mind is associated, the Yogi is transformed as it were, into that!" **-Adi Shankaracharya, *Vivekachudamani*, 369-370 (Swami Madhavananda Translation)**

References:

1. http://en.wikipedia.org/wiki/Ian_Stevenson

2. http://en.wikipedia.org/wiki/Psychological_astrology#Jungian_legacy

Bibliography:

Karma in Yoga and Ayurveda: *Durgadas (Rodney) Lingham: Academy of Traditional Ayurveda, 2013*

Satyarth Prakash: *Maharishi Dayananda Saraswati*

Classical Texts:

Charaka Samhita

Sushruta Samhita

Sharngadhara Samhita

Ashtanga Hridayam

Madhava Nidana

Rig Veda Samhita

Brihadaranyaka Upanishad

Shatapatha Brahmana

Vivekachudamani

Bhava Prakasha

VIII. Conclusion:

While some may be unhappy with the approach taken here, it is validated by both tradition as well as the *Samhitas*. While the BAMS (Bachelor of Ayurvedic Medicine and Surgery) is often attacked, the mainstream texts in the south have been *Ashtanga Hridaya* and others, itself which combines the traditions of
both *Charaka* and *Sushruta* and hence looks back to an age of synthesis, while also not forgetting the traditional and spiritual aspects of Ayurveda, that still remain alive and well in the South today, alongside traditions lost in the North, such
as *Kalari* (Vedic *Dhanurveda* or martial arts), the system of manipulation of *marmas* to temporarily stop the flow of blood, place a patient into a coma and so forth, which is a dangerous art but nonetheless, originated with *Sushrutacharya* and his unique ability to both heal these and manipulate them.

I am not against the modern *marma* therapies, but only against their dangers. One must first harness the powers of *Pranashakti* and also know deeply how the *marmas* operate before manipulating them. In *Kerala* also, exist the Ayurveda of the *Thiyya* school of *Kalari* masters, former nurses and masseurs or therapists in Ayurveda that incorporated their non-*Samhita* based styles (for they were considered low to outcasts as originally *Sinhalese* Buddhist monks).

As we have noted, Ayurveda is far older than the *Atharvaveda* it is said to have come from. Eye-transplants, head-transplants, skin-rejuvenation and others were performed as early as the *Rig Veda*.

Yet, on another level apart from the physical state, the Vedic Ayurveda was one of mantras, as it understood the root-causes of viruses and bacteria physically were negative astral entities and for diseases, were karmic factors. The later Vedic *Yajna* itself is a physical manifestation of the inner psycho-physical workings of the biological *doshas* etc. in the body and spiritual powers and workings of the inner causal and subtle bodies.

Thus, the hymns worked as *prayaschitta* (atonement) and to ward off the negative harmful astral forces (*rakshasagrahas*) behind physical ones. These mantras contained special powers through rhythms etc. which even united fractured bones, treated insanity, cancer etc. by working first on the subtle body, repairing it and hence then the physical. This is a deeper side of working with the *shakti* healing, that went along with various powers of the hymns and their metres themselves.

As noted, the greater Ayurveda considers wrongful diet and incompatible foods to create *manovahasrota mala-vyadhi* (vitiation of toxins in the mental channels), causing *prajnaparadha* (vitiation of the intellect), leading to *adharmic* karmas (unrighteous actions) which give birth to *papakarmas* or negative karmas (or karmic residue, *sanskaras*), stored in the *chitta* or mind-consciousness and continues onto the next body through reincarnation (*samsara*). As a result of these challenges, *sahaja* (congenital) factors affect the embryo in *janma* (genetic manners) of either *matrija* (maternal) or *pitrija* (paternal) sides, relating to the subtle cause of genetic factors, which are often *asadhya* (incurable). Charaka Rishi describes *arshas* (piles) and *prameha* (diabetes) of genetic varieties.

Hence why methods to rectify one's karma or DNA at a subtle level is most important, as the mantras of the Vedic period address, to properly heal the causative factors behind congenital disorders.

The *Atharvaveda* and the *Rig Veda* thus contain several healing mantras. *Atharvaveda* (IV.12) mentions such mantras to help unite bones and fractures, which are perhaps mantric techniques used by the *Ashwins* to restore heads and limbs when severed. Gemstone-mantra charms as in *Atharvaveda* (VIII.5) as also others for invocation of deities and forces to ward of various diseases as well as germs, viruses or bacteria (VIII.6) are also common. Healing with *Prana* or life-force through the hands is also mentioned (*Atharvaveda*, IV.13). This older *mantric Ayurveda* of the *Rig Veda* grew into the *Atharvaveda* and hence preceded what later became surgical techniques, by first empowering herbs and substances, as we also see in *Atharvaveda*.

In ancient times, certain *astra-chikitsa mantras* or healing weapon-chants were done to heal wounds, restore fractures and such, in older ages (*yugas*), which are said to be more spiritual. It was through this that the science of surgery itself arose, from subtle techniques, via the *Ashwin* gods, as noted.

The scope of Ayurveda as also in recognising these subtle factors behind the physical disorders and encompassing and embracing them is hence a model that can be researched East and West in the future.

We have noted *Charaka's* statement about *Vishavayu,* meaning toxic or poisonous air, which also relates to the *tanmatra* or touch and the skin, meaning also impressions that are absorbed via the skin as toxins that can produce diseases as well as entering the *prana* or oxygen and life-force within us through breath. Simple *Agni-Hotras* were a traditionally effective way to remove these and on a subtle level, airborne bacteria are derived from harmful negative energies in the elements (*rakshasa-bhuta*) in Vedic thought, which the mantras help dispel. Just as the *doshas* or biological humours in the body can become unbalanced, so also the energies in our surroundings can relative to the elements and hence *Vastu* (Vedic Feng Shui) mantras to the directions and deities can help restore these to balance at a subtle level.

As we know, in ancient non-Abrahamic cultures, there exist a variety of transcendental (*para*), greater celestial (*mahadeva*), celestial seers (*rishi*) as also celestial (*deva*), lower celestial (*upadeva*) as celestial nymphs and musicians as *apsaras, gandharvas, kinnaras* etc. and also several classes of semi-divine beings, such as serpentine beings (*nagas*), tree-dwellers and guardians of underground wealth (*yakshas*) as well as various classes of spirits and ghouls such as *pretas, bhutas, vetalas* and *pishachas* and then various classes of negative astral entities, which include the *asura, rakshasa, brahma-rakshasa, daitya* and *danava* etc. These are often said to cross over into the human plane at times and even possess subtle *vimanas* or airships that can manifest themselves. Usually however, their presence around humans is of a subtle, even nefarious nature, simply to afflict suffering, pain and be a general nuisance to humanity and higher beings. For this reason, the ancient *Vedic* texts contain hymns and sacred rituals to dispel these from our presence and environments and bring down the grace of the higher, even *para* or transcendental deities, reflecting the later wrathful forms of the

Divine in Hinduism, forms of the deity Shiva and the Goddess, *Shakti*, the celestial power of the cosmos itself. Sometimes even the *Devas* or celestials must collectively invoke them from the higher transcendental worlds to destroy powerful causal-bodied negative entities, such as *brahma-rakshasas* (powerful demons who were once *Brahmins* or priests and become demonic in the afterlife) and the titans, or *daityas* and *danavas*. The Ayurvedic classics are quite clear about these entities and their influences also.

The *Atharvaveda* itself credits many diseases due to negative astral forces of several varieties, which produce *bhutas* (elemental parasites, viruses or bacteria) also known as *krimi* or viruses etc. that become airborne through the elements (*bhutas*) of wind, water etc. and travel. Ancient cultures not only in India, but also ancient Tibet, China and the Americas as other shaman and native faiths also had a sophisticated knowledge of the actual root-causes of bacteria and viruses, not simply their physical manifestation (*vyakta*) stage as allopathy focuses on and hence looked at these subtle origins and elimination of root-causes behind them, which could often also be karmic in nature (due to *adharmika karmas* or unrighteous actions in past lives). Other cultures also had their special amulets and prayers or hymns to bring in the higher Divine Powers of Light to combat the lower forces of Darkness that were behind disease. These are not simply imaginary or far-fetched ideas, for the ancients, as noted, also realised there were airborne bacteria and physical or exogenous causes for diseases, but these parasites were produced or had their origin from the subtle non-physical negative entities.

We need to take these into consideration in our world today to really be effective in treating disease, but along with this, also realise the scope and depth of surgery that Ayurveda itself has given us, and also the original rules relating to surgical conduct and healing of wounds, care of the patient and subtle and physical factors relating to these, which are often ignored in the modern world and modern medical science, again, East and West!

Likewise, the various depth of Ayurveda and what it has given modern surgery and surpassed it has also been flung into oblivion in favour of the radical views of promotion of spiritual Ayurveda which, while having its place, even in *Charaka*'s internal medicine school, also employs the use of surgery. Yet, modern medical science should also not underestimate the power of karmic afflictions in both causing diseases and complicating these, and one cannot simply rectify these by surgery or rational therapies alone.

For this reason, I propose, as in my book **Purna Ayurveda Pariksha**, a complete system of Ayurveda, bringing in all aspects and facets of the Yoga science, from Vedanta to Tantra, of ritualism, of *Jyotisha* or astrology of varied types, including *Anka Jyotisha* (numerology) and *Samudrika Shastra* (palmistry and face-reading), expanded aspects of *Mahabhuta* and *Graha* (planetary) etc. types of *Prakriti* beyond the *tridosha* as discussed, as also *Vastu Shastra* and so on, all of which have sanction in the sacred texts of Ayurveda which, albeit redacted several times (*Ashwini Samhita* predated *Agnivesha Tantra* which was a precursor to *Charaka Samhita* etc.), still contains the *bijas* or seeds and origins of what once was, a more complete, integral and advanced system of Ayurveda that we can restore today in all respects, just as *Dridhbala* had the vision, working from older texts, to reconstruct the *Charaka*

Samhita from older texts existing at his time of the *Atreya sampradaya*, so that the greater wisdom of Ayurveda would not be lost to the tests of time!

Namah Shivaya!

Charaka Mantra:
Om Cham Charakaya Namaha!

Charaka Gayatri:
Om Tat Purushaya Vidmahe,
Vasudevaya Dhimahi,
Tanno Charakah Prachodayat!

Sushruta Gayatri:
Om Tat Purushaya Vidmahe,
Vishwamitraputraya Dhimahi,
Tanno Sushrutah Prachodayat!

Endnotes:

1. Dr. B.R. Suhas, *Sushruta*, Sapna Book House, Bangalore, 2011

2. Studies have shown that Lesbians are more likely to suffer from polycystic ovaries and ovarian cancer than heterosexual women. Some cases also cite breast Cancer more likely and on this, Charaka also continues that these females are born without breasts (noting the possible loss of them due to breast cancer in ancient times), as also Vata vitiating and destroying the ovaries. Sources:
(i) http://www.ncbi.nlm.nih.gov/pubmed/15533359 (ii) http://www.dailymail.co.uk/health/article-186777/Lesbian-link-PCOS.html

3. Note traditional sources as below:

i. Article on Tantra and its Misconceptions, with special reference to chakras and their distorted modern perceptions by Dr. David Frawley (Pandit Vamadeva Shastri):

http://vedanet.com/2012/06/13/tantra-and-its-misconceptions-reclaiming-the-essence-from-the-illusions/

ii. Section on Chakras from **"From the River of Heaven"** by Dr. David Frawley (Pandit Vamadeva Shastri) and note on limited use of modern-day chakra-balancing compared to inner Yoga and *Jnana* and *Bhakti* concerns re chakras

iii. **"Ayurveda and the Mind"** by Dr. David Frawley (Pandit Vamadeva Shastri) (p.312-313) which stresses the New Age distortions confusing the inner with outer concerns of chakras and psychological states and derangements

iv. **"Ayurvedic Healing"** by Dr. David Frawley (Pandit Vamadeva Shastri) (p. 334-335) in which he references meditational, pranayama and meditational disorders which again stresses the traditional all-encompassing rather than modern limited view of *Kundalini*, Yoga techniques etc. and their dangers and cautions traditionally

v. **"Yoga and Ayurveda"** by Dr. David Frawley (Pandit Vamadeva Shastri) (p. 138-141) stresses also the dangers of playing with chakras and mistake of New Age healers and chakra workings seeing and working on them as physical in the body

vi. **"Tantric Yoga and the Wisdom Goddesses"** by Dr. David Frawley (Pandit Vamadeva Shastri), (p.179-181), stressing of the New Age distortions of the chakras also.

vii. In his book **"Kundalini Yoga"**, under 'The Gradual Ascent of the Mind', Swami Sivananda also states on chakras:

"The Chakras are centres of Shakti as vital force—in other words, these are centres of Pranashakti manifested by Pranavayu in the living body, the presiding Devatas of which

are the names for the Universal Consciousness as it manifests in the form of these centres. The Chakras are not perceptible in the gross senses. Even if they were perceptible in the living body which they help to organise they disappear with the disintegration of organism at death."

viii. The great Yogi, Swami Yogeshwaranand Paramhansa has stated in his book "**Atma Vijnana**" (p. 69) that the chakras are not physical as some writers have stated and is incorrect that they are physical structures as:

"...these structures are not perceived without special meditation, nor can their activity be equated with their gross structure."

He continues *"...it is not enough simply to perceive these chakra-s. One must experience directly position and movement of the Prana-s (vital airs) which pervades the chakra-s; one must experience their colours, forms and functions of the Prana-s and the five Tanmatra-s (subtle elements) implied within them."*

4. Recent investigations have shown that *Saraswata Churna*, an ancient preparation used to enhance the mind and treat a variety of psychological disorders, was as effective as Citalopram in treating Geriatric Depression. Source: http://www.jourlib.org/paper/2338130#.VPzWGXyUdu4 / http://www.irjponline.com/admin/php/uploads/vol-2_issue-6/16.pdf

5. Commonly used in southern India in treating mental disorders, studies have shown that *Manasamitra Vataka* is effective in treating General Anxiety Disorder, along with *Shirodhara* (medicated pouring of oil on the head) and hence reveals Ayurvedic medications have potentials for proving safer and natural alternatives to biochemical drugs in treating such disorders.
Source: http://www.researchgate.net/publication/229073616_Clinical_efficacy_of_Manasamitra_Vataka_%28an_Ayurveda_medication%29_on_generalized_anxiety_disorder_with_comorbid_generalized_social_phobia_a_randomized_controlled_study

6. Beneficial results of honey are seen in weight loss and blood lipids in diabetic patients: Source: http://www.ncbi.nlm.nih.gov/pubmed/19817641

Further Discussions on Ayurveda's Science and New-Age Misconceptions:

I. Ayurvedic Microbiology: *An Historical Examination*

Background:

Ayurvedic microbiology goes back to the Rig Veda where these parasites were known as *rakshasas* ("those who injure"), which their elaboration of numerous types being identified in the *Atharvaveda* - VIII.6) around 3000BCE, where numerous parasites were seen as causing diseases - many of them were seen to cause derangements in the breaths or pranas entering the body.

Around the 6th Century BC, the Jainas described the "*Nigodas*", which were a microorganism and lowest form of life causing diseases and living in certain plants, atmosphere etc. Ayurvedic texts describe these entities as being from the size of a sesame seed to even extremely minute (*sukshma*) or unseen by the human eye (*Madhava Nidana*, VII.11-12). They form in the stomach, sometimes as worms and other times as subtle parasites entering the bloodstream (*raktavahasrotas*) (ibid, *Charaka, Vimanasthana,* VII.11). In such cases they can eat away skin, blood-vessels, sinews, ligaments etc. Ayurvedic Classics give many types that can cause schizophrenia or insanity (*unmada*), headaches (*siroroga*), heart disease (*hridroga*), tooth decay (*dantaroga*) as well as other medical problems.

The *Rig Veda* (5000BCE) describes their first manifestation as causing disease as well as their destruction via light:

"***The shining light (deva) expels all the rakshasas and yatudhanas, with all those offensive defects (prati-dosham, Vikriti) and hatred.***"
- Rig Veda. I.35.10

Rakshasas are those who injure, destroy etc. *Yatudhanas* are another class of *rakshasas*. *Yatudhana* comes from *yatu* (to attack) and *dhana* (to hold or contain). They are thus parasites that attack and hold disease within the body. *Prati-dosham* can also mean the "offensive vitiation / defect", *dosha* meaning 'defect' and a synonym for disease.

Cancer and Microbial Lifeforms:

The Sanskrit term *arbuda* (one hundred million, swelling) also identified the one hundred million cancer cells today; parasites entering the bloodstream in Ayurveda are also identified as formally mentioned, thus also giving rise to certain disorders such as blood cancer (*raktarbuda - Madhava Nidana*, XXXVIII.20-21).

The 5th Century Physician *Vagbhata* in his *Ashtanga Hridaya* (*Uttarasthana, 29*), mentions other causes of Cancer as follows:

(i) *Malas* or wastes created from *kapha* (phlegm or excess protein) entering into the tissues and causing swelling and growths

(ii) *Rakta* or blood-cancer (Leukaemia) are caused by aggravated *doshas* that cause parasites (*krimi* - Leukemia cells) which invades veins and muscles etc.

(iii) Muscular tumours result due to excess eating of meats (also *Bhava Prakasha, Madhya Khanda, III.44.22-23 / Madhava Nidana, XXXVIII.22-23*)

(iv) Fatty tumours as a result of excess foods with too much fatty substance, which moves to the muscles and skin causing tumours

(v) Bone cancer develops as a result of fractures and injuries

Likewise, *Madhava* states that:

(vi) Secondary cancers or malignant tumours occur along with the first, causing incurability of cancer (*Madhava Nidana, XXXVIII.25*)

(vii) Expanding on with regards to *mamasarbuda* or cancer of the muscle-tissue, such can also be caused by injuries from fighting etc. that over a period of time give rise to a cancerous tumour (*Madhava Nidana, XXXVIII.22-23*, also *Sushruta, Nidanasthana, XI.17-18*)

Later texts state such as surgery, cauterisation and alkalis are the therapies. *Sushruta Samhita (Nidana, XI.15-16); Madhava Nidana* (XXXVIII.2) etc. also state that *vata* (wind) and other *doshas* increase in the body and bring about abnormalities in the blood, muscles and fat that cause tumours. *Charaka Samhita*(XVIII.33) also states that tumours or cancer is classified under a type of swelling and treated accordingly. This would also agree with the Vedic ideal of cancers being *apachi* or swellings and also malignant tumours (*arbuda*).
Charaka (Chikitsasthana), 12, 81-87 also states that Cancer is to be treated like tumours (malignant) by removal etc. *Vagbhata* (5th Century) mentions cancers be treated afterwards by *ksharas* and *agnikarma* - alkalis and cauterisation (*Ashtanga Hridaya, Sutrasthana*, 30.3 & 42). Such ideas go back to the *Rig Veda* (X.67.12), where cauterisation or destruction by electrical force was applied to destroy cancerous tumours after they were cut off (*arbuda* - cancer; *indra* = *vidyut* or electrical current / energy / lightening).

The importance of this is also well-stated in the ancient Hindu *shastras*; such texts also warn that the entire tumour should be removed without leaving any residue, otherwise it can (potentially) kill the patient - here using the analogy of fire (by a spark).(*Sushruta Samhita, Chikitsasthana*, XVIII.42).

Classical texts also speak of comprehensive manners in which to heal and seal the wound and purify it after these procedures to stop re-occurrence of the tumours and also heal the wounds. These are done according to the *dosha* (classified vitiation) involved.

Sound Therapies and Microorganisms:

Sushruta Samhita also has *mantras* with various frequencies or sounds and special fumigation rituals to help protect against them, especially post-surgery, where they are seen to attack a person whose wounds are exposed or ulcerating, thus perhaps also the cause behind cancers manifesting today from cysts removed and surgeries - the term used again is *rakshasa* (those which injure). *Sushruta (Sutrasthana, XIX.27)* here makes note of mustard, neem, ghee and salt used to fumigate the area of the wounded to keep away any bacteria that may enter during the night (*nishachara*).

The chanting of *mantras* here daily according to Vedic rhythms is hence also noted, as such perhaps have frequencies that penetrate the sub-molecular levels of the ethers (hence *akshara* - *Sanskrit* syllable which relates to *akasha* - ether) at the level of the *paramanu* (subatomic level) in *Vaisheshika* (Hindu physics), thus dispelling or creating frequencies that keep these minute parasites at bay (similar to frequencies heard by dogs by unheard by humans). The knowledge of the ancients in *Sanskrit* is not unknown; the *Chandahshastra* by *Pingala* (500BCE) dealing with Vedic metres used the world's first binary numeral system and contains Fibonacci numbers.

Aryabhatta's numeral system involving letters of the Sanskrit alphabet or *aksharas* (5th Century) and the Vedic study of *shabdas* or sounds of each letter of the Sanskrit alphabet along with the world's oldest grammarian, *Panini* (600BCE) also testify to the scientific nature of the Sanskrit language employed as an artificial language from antiquity.

The Kashmiri *Spanda Karikas* also expand on such ideas, relative to the atomic formation of the world - here emanating from the primal *spanda* (vibration) connected to sound. Here the letters of the *Sanskrit* alphabet becomes forms of the primal *spandashakti* (vibratory power) of creation itself, seen as rays of the Goddess from the transcendental sound or the *bindu* (*shakti*, the vibratory power-sound of the Goddess) emanating the rays giving birth to elements in the following order: cosmic mind - 64 rays, ether / manifest sound - 72 rays, air / primal friction - 54 rays, heat or form - 62 rays, water or taste perception - 52 rays and earth / solid matter or smell - 56 rays, totally 360 (*Saundarya Lahari, XIV*).

The paratomic (*paramanu* or sub-atomic) effect of *Sanskrit aksharas* or syllables examined and formed into words or sacred chants (*mantras*) can be understood by the term *mantra* (from *manas* - "mind" + *tra* - that "which takes beyond"); the Hindu system of physics of *Vaisheshika* around 800BCE (Yogananda, Autobiography of a Yogi), measures the mind as an atom in nature- "*The mind is atomic in nature*". (*Vaisheshika Sutras* VII.1.30).

The integral system of physics / atomism within Ayurveda as an integral system should also not be forgotten. *Charaka (Charaka Samhita Sharirasthana*, VII.17) also cites such views, stating that *paramanus* (sub-atomic particles) form the basis of the body's most subtle (*sauksmika*) composition and their union and de-materialisation are both due to *vayu* (wind, the force of action, motion or movement etc.); *Charaka* here stating this after mentioning the *mahabhutas* (great elements, viz. ether, air, fire, water and earth) in the body, giving rise to its formation. A similar idea is expressed in the *Brihadaranyaka Upanishad,* IV.2.3, where minute arteries are described as so fine as 1/1000th of a human hair!

Such methods may seem far-fetched however, yet we should not forget that our decimal system and numerals (0 to 9) replacing the cumbersome Roman system came from

India, as out concept of zero, trigonometrical functions, the origin of calculus, algebra, quadratic equations etc.

Anti-Parasitical Methods and Post-Operative Procedures:

While we have discussed the effects of sound-therapies and the importance of various techniques in dispelling harmful microorganisms, the complex surgical methods in Ayurveda are often thought to have little value.

However, by contrast, ancient methods after operative procedures (*Charaka Samhita, Chikitsasthan*a, XXV, 101-106) included *agnikarma* (thermal cauterisation) or *kshara* (alkali cauterisation) of the area, followed by pouring hot ghee or bee's wax on the area and suturing, which prevented air or bacteria getting into the wound, as well as placing the patient in a specially fumigated room or chamber, where hymns were chanted etc. to prevent or ward off negative entities causing physical airborne bacteria. Ancient post-operative procedures were hence much more advanced than today's practices!
Abhisanga-jwara or fever for example, caused by lust (*kama*), grief (*shoka*), fear (*bhaya*) or anger (*krodha*) or *abhishakta* (harmful microorganisms) in *Charaka Samhita* (*Chikitsasthana*, III.114-117) is also related to poisonous air and *bhutas* (negative astral entities). Here, the mental factors are causative, the *bhutas* or microorganisms or negative entities they cause, which hence vitiate the air or environment, causing such fevers and diseases. The primal causes however are past-life factors and deeds or actions which bring them about in the person (*Charaka, Chikitsa*, III.13-14) - citing not mere random fate, but the logical system of *karana-karya* or cause and effect in Ayurveda.
These ancient methods are hence much more complex than today for surgery and also require the patient undergo specific diets, regime and rest for rejuvenation afterwards, which is often not done today. Even the care of the wounds today, let alone bedside manner, is contradictory to the time of the great Ayurvedic physicians, which is no wonder cancer has become almost impossible to cure in conventional medicine!

It also here considers that the ancient Ayurvedic physicians, relative to the knowledge of microbiology, also consider the cause and further threat of cancer to be fueled by these airborne parasites, even if they were of different varieties from the causative pathogen.
Bhava Prakasha (*Madhya Khand*a, 52.49) on contagious skin diseases also lists fevers, ulcers and specifically *Bhutonmada* (insanity caused by *bhutas* or supernatural forces / elements, as noted here) to be passed on through sexual intercourse, breath (i.e airborne bacteria or viruses specifically – Ayurvedic texts list *krimi* as parasites directly from clothes, sharing foods etc. of infected people. Hence, this also confirms again these are bacteria and viruses.

Relative to psychology, these parasites were known as *graha* (those which grab hold or seize) and *bhuta* (element - i.e., those which enter via elemental forces of nature - airborne, water, solids as foods etc.). On this, *Charaka* (*Charaka Samhit*a, *Sutrasthana*, XI.45) clarifies that *Bhuta*-caused means the elements - viz. *vishavayu* (poisoned air), *agni* (fire and heat) etc.and *manasa* (mentally-caused) are due to emotional upsets etc. as unfulfilled desires.

The ancient Physician *Charaka* (*Charaka Samhita, Sutrasthana,* XXX.13-14) states that in order to preserve vitality (*ojas*) in the body, one should avoid mental afflictions and make sure one's *srotas* (bodily channels) are cleansed and calm for knowledge (*jnana*). This would imply that psychological issues that are karmic or deep-seated are behind the *karana-nidana* or causal origin of the cancer itself in the Vedic philosophy. It is certainly the opinion of the *Atharva Veda*, from which Ayurveda itself originates (*Charaka Samhita, Sutrasthana, XXX.21)* that many diseases are caused by parasites and primary (first measure) of treatment is the spiritual (mental as we shall discuss) along with herbal measures.

The 20 types mentioned in *Sarngadhara Samhita* hence have their origins here. *Krityonmada,* caused by rituals etc. would be due to trying to perform actions to gain wealth, [belief or delusion that one has] supernatural powers etc. and due to a failure of such, one falls into insanity (as in cases of anxiety-depression etc.). Curse of a Guru can be described as (a) karmic, but also a result of one's Guru or teacher chastising them or (b) taking away titles and positions of the disciple, causing grief and hence mental agony causing depression - similar to what we have noted relative to microorganisms and tribes of people by their karmic effects or physical insults causing mania (logically speaking - we will discuss karma further on). *Sushruta* (*Sushruta Samhit*a, Uttarasthana, LX.5) states that these *grahas* (*bhutas*) enter a person who is wounded or not, unclean in habits (inferring bacteria) etc. which also reveals these as airborne bacteria and subject to external toxins, viruses and so forth. He also states (*Uttarasthana*, LX.37), that if they do not go away by chanting of mantras etc. (sound-effects and spiritual therapies for the mind or Psycho-therapy), then they should be treated with medical drugs.

Charaka (*Charaka Samhita, Sutrasthana,* XI.46, 54) states of these therapies, that they are there to keep the mind freed of unwholesome objects (or from performing bad actions, further complicating the disease) and hence their employment in treatment (*mano-nigraha* - attempts to subdue the mind), which constitutes *Sattvavajaya* or psychological therapies - of which *Daivavyapashraya*, the "illuminating therapies" or psycho-somatic / placebo therapies hence form an integral part of and are done along with *Yuktivyapashraya*, that is, rational therapies as diet, herbs and formulas for the mind.

"Shock-therapies" were also given in various cases according to the specific mental derangement also. *Charaka* thus states that opposite therapies according to the mental disorder (*Charaka Samhita, Sutrasthana,* XI.46) should be adopted, which proves such "spiritual therapies" were mental distractions and psychological tools for also providing detachment of the mind, mental disorder etc. *Charaka* (*Chikitsasthana*, IX.96) also states that insanity can be avoided if one abstains from eating meats and wines or impure diets etc. and hence seen as causative factors (*nidanas*) of various kinds of insanity. Various meats and also alcohol are given various factors or qualities (*gunas*) in Ayurveda, according to their chemical reactions upon the mind, which are described as aggravating *rajas* and *tamas* in the mental channels, blurring our perceptions - relative again to parasites caused in the bloodstream by bad diet etc. and this producing chemical imbalances in the brain, similar to dream-substance:

"Bad dreams occur due to the blockages in the manovahasrotas (mind carrying

channels), due to aggravated wastes (malas) in the body."
-Ashtanga Hridaya, Sharirasthana,VI.59-60

Charaka Samhita (Nidanasthana, VII.4) also states this, citing the causative factor as unclean foods, distressed minds etc. and bad dietary regimes, bad postures as even mental factors such as passion, anger, greed, fear, confusion, grief, anxiety etc. that causes the mind to become unstable and causes *doshas* or the vitiations to spread into the mental channels going into the brain through the bloodstream from the heart, causing psychosis.

As with *Charaka, Sushruta* takes this rational approach *(Sutrasthana,* I.25) and states that *manasika* (psychic) disorders are caused
by *krodha* (anger), *shoka* (grief), *bhaya* (fear), *harsha* (exhilaration), *vishada* (sadness), *k ama* (lust), *lobha* (greed) etc. and similarly, *Madhava Nidana* (XX.14-15) states insanity is brought on my fright, loss of wealth, death of family members, excessive sexual desire etc. which also further infers these are due to mutations, issues etc. of these various organs.

On this note, Ayurveda gives various properties to foods based upon their respective effects upon the *manas* (mind) and the *deha* (body), relative to (a) their *aharashakti* (digestive power or ability to be metabolised) and (b) their ability to agitate or dull the mind through their *tikshna* (penetrating and thus irritating) or *manda* (low and dull) quality when entering the bloodstream and hence are the root-causative factors of all diseases, both psychic and somatic (*Charaka Samhita, Sutrsthana,* XXVIII.45-48). Here, the effects of *rasa* (taste) upon the biological humours in the body, the *virya* (potency) and thereby *vipaka* (post-metabolised effect) are ascertained for each herb or food; Ayurvedic classics here give different properties for example within sub-groups of even honies and sugars here and their specific effects as also curative effects upon diseases, let alone the body and mind, employing the system,as per one's *Prakriti-dosha* (natural constitutional nature) and *Vikara* (vitiation or diseased stated), age, sex, climate and season, not all foods, dietary regimes and energetics are good for one and all as a generic system and can also produce diseases!

In addition, what vitiates the mind and body as also parasites in the external and internal bodily wastes, the blood, mucus in the stomach and also in the feces due to the latter by parasites in the GI tract (*Charaka Samhita, Vimanasthana,* VII.9-14), is also due to (a) incompatible food combinations and (b) wrong *ahara* (diet), *vyayama* (exercise) and other lifestyle regimes (drinking, smoking, excess worry etc. causing slow or variable metabolism, causing *ama* or toxins in the digestive system, which then spread throughout the body).

*Sushruta (Uttarasthana, LIV.*1-7) lists the exact causes of parasites in the body as arising from dirty foods, lack of exercise, hard to digest foods - especially flour, pulses, leafy greens, vinegar, curd, milk (hence excess dairy), jaggery and sugarcane juice (sugars), tahini, fried foods, sweet and sour drinks and animals from marshy regions. Before giving treatments, he notes seven categories of these blood-parasites (*raktaja krimi)* - ibid, 15-16.

Conclusion:

There are many advanced concepts in the *Ayurvedic* texts. *Charaka* and *Sushruta* around 1500BCE for example describe two types of diabetes - Type 1 characterised by genetic factors (*sahaja*) due to vitiation in the genetic seed from either mother or father and Type 2, characterised by obesity.

In addition, *Sushruta Samhita* with rhinoplasty and otoplasty methods that were adopted during the British Raj in southern India during the Mysore Wars and taken to England by the surgeon Joseph Constantine Carpue and still employed today by plastic surgeons have contributed to modern medical procedures. The novel use of large ants as surgical clips by *Sushruta* is also well-known for perforated bowels.

In his translation of the *Sushruta Samhita* (XIV.18), the erudite Ayurvedic *vaidya* and scholar, SR Srikantha Murthy (published by Chaukhambha Orientalia, Varanasi, 2007) notes:

"The above description of surgical operation of the abdomen laboratory and intestinal loop (enterotomy) is a testimony for the progress achieved by the surgeons of ancient India. Making use of big ants to hold the tissues is a novel method and a precedent of the use of clips used now- a- days. Mixture of honey and ghee as a preventative against sepsis - has been recently proved by medical researchers of Japan (sic)". (Vol III, p.148).

He similarly makes a note of the puncturing the abdomen and draining of fluids by the ancient Hindu physicians by the same method in the modern day (ibid, p.149). *Sushruta* states that there are 1120 diseases that plague man and 573 drugs that have been enumerated in his treatise (*Sushruta, Uttarasthana,* LXVI.7-9). Of diseases, there are said to be 62 combinations of the *doshas* (ibid, 10-2) and *asamkhyeya* (innumerable) when combining when the bodily tissues and wastes (ibid, 12-13).

As such, we have established the deep knowledge of the ancients in the fields of medicine, especially in microbiology from the earliest Vedic times down to the present-day through Ayurveda. There are also methods described (such as the employment of *mantras*) of which requires further study today, as also the other methods of ancient times such as applications of alkalis and various herbal compounds on wounds for their purification and healing that are largely ignored today, as well as the methods of fumigation and others. Mustard and neem for example both have antiseptic properties and were used for fumigation, as well as ghee and salt which is an interesting combination with the former.

The ancient use of ghee and honey for example, described in the ancient texts has proven useful in studies for their ability of healing wounds and has shown to inhibit bacteria [1]. Such examples are also testimony of the ancient knowledge of microbiology / parasitology and provide examples of effects for the future, making us question many of our modern methods and their actual efficiency!

As an example, *Ayurvedic Dinacharya* (daily regimes) included the following:

Oral care by way of tooth cleaning, oil-pulling, tongue-scraping, betel-chewing, oleation of the nostrils (to avoid mucous in sinuses and sinus-related issues) and ears (to improve hearing and reduce excess build up of wax, issues such as tinnitus etc.), moderate (not forced) exercise, stressing the effects of under and over-exercise in disease (as also wrongful and forced positions as in modern yoga), washing the face with Indian gooseberry and cold water for good complexion, applying collyrium to the eyes for stronger eyesight as well as massage of and care of the feet (by wearing shoes) to also prevent eye-troubles, massaging the head with oil to prevent falling and greying of the hairs as well as bodily oleation (massage) to promote strength, good circulation and complexion, trimming nails, hair on the beard, public area etc. (to prevent any germs etc. being lodged in such areas), correct exposure to sunlight to improve metabolism (or to cool breezes when metabolism is excessive), having proper sleep and engaging in proper conduct (as avoiding gambling, alcoholism, avoiding joining organisations or second-hand clothing, jewellery etc.).

In addition, various seasonal regimes (*ritucharyas*) were also employed along with proper intake of liquids, foods (*ahara*) and combinations suitable for one's age, sex, location, climate and seasons is also conducive to avoiding diseases - naturally however those such as *sahaja / atmaja* (congenital) become more difficult, but by reducing such impressions down, diseases such as cancer and severe parasitical disorders as we suffer from today, as also psychic, can be overcome as we have discussed by examples earlier. For above all, many diseases in modern allopathy and Ayurveda alike are caused by bacteria entering the body and are the cause of our intake of various drugs to eliminate them which can be avoided and supplements taken that directly target and eliminate them (such as turmeric, *neem* - Azadirachta indica, licorice, *kushta* - Saussurea costus, *manjishtha* - Rubia cordifolia, honey etc.) as also those which help rejuvenate our bodies such as *amalaki* (Emblica indica), *bhringaraja* (Eclipta alba), *ashwagandha* (Withania somnifera), *bala* (Sida cordifolia), *shilajit*(ashphaltum), *guduchi* (Tinospora cordifolia) etc.

Footnotes / References:

1. http://www.ncbi.nlm.nih.gov/pmc/articles/PMC3144338/

Research Bibliography:

Ashtanga Hridayam - Translation by K.R Srikantha Murthy, Chaukhambha Orientalia, Varanasi

Charaka Samhita - Translation by K.R Srikantha Murthy, Chaukhambha Orientalia, Varanasi

Sushruta Samhita - Translation by K.R Srikantha Murthy, Chaukhambha Orientalia, Varanasi

Sarngadhara Samhita - Translation by K.R Srikantha Murthy, Chaukhambha Orientalia, Varanasi

Madhava Nidana - Translation by K.R Srikantha Murthy, Chaukhambha Orientalia,

Varanasi

Bhava Prakasha - Translation by K.R Srikantha Murthy, Chaukhambha Orientalia, Varanasi

Purna Ayurveda Pariksha: Durgadas (Rodney) Lingham

The Complexity of Charaka's Ayurveda: Durgadas (Rodney) Lingham

Arya Nyaya Vijnana: Durgadas (Rodney) Lingham

Rig Veda Samhita

Atharva Veda

Brihadaranyaka Upanishad

Vaisheshika Sutras

Saundarya Lahiri of Sri Shankaracharya

II. Baseless Claims of Reiki and Pranic Healing

Have you ever thought about or have you ever experienced Reiki and similar methods such as *chakra*-balancing and *Pranic Healing*? <u>Did you know that there is no traditional basis to such methods?</u>

Today we embrace the period of *Kali-Yuga*, the age of decline in culture and civilisation. However in the modern world, we wish to take highly advanced and developed concepts from the ancient masters, within whose traditions such were tailored as per individuals and also took traditional teachers and spiritual aspirants (*sadhakas*) born in native soil and within native traditions, and make them our own - applying them often to "healing" and "mental health". Good examples here are meditation, Yoga and others such as the systems of Reiki and Pranic Healing, which have recently been developed.

Traditionally in India, *Pranic Healing* didn't involve the laying of hands, crystals and other such that the modern post-Christian world still with Christian subliminal *samskaras* embraces not in the traditional scientific and rational manner, but in the "magical" and "unexplained" manner such is adopted and epitomised by the naivety of the European mind and its zeal to take such "half truths" and zealously proselytise them! *Pranic Healing* in India in Yoga groups went no further than *Pranayama*, the various breathing techniques in Yoga by which toxic air is thrown from the body and the biological humours or "faults" (*doshas*) were reduced or increased accordingly, as per the physical application of such breathing practices and their biological effects, as also by oxygenating the blood.

Such of course is quite different to the modern methods of "laying hands" that appears to represent a more Pentecostal approach that has superimposed itself upon eastern healing modalities. While ancient Yogis in India, as in China could manipulate the *Prana* or *Qi* within a patient's body, such wasn't done by laying or hands, but by the influence of their minds or the effect of their own pure *prana* or life-force developed through severe austerities, disciplines and training; such traditional *Vaidyas* or Ayurvedic Physicians could heal a person by *drishti* (sight) or their presence alone - some did impart it by *sparsha* (touch), but such was not merely superficial and usually involved a mere short touch of a person - though such was not necessary and was more or less for the benefit of the receiver alone. And again, such is far different to the so-called methods of "energy transferal" imparted by people belonging to no actual tradition, having no Guru or lineage to connect to and devoid of any true spiritual practices, austerities or knowledge of greater systems of Yoga and *Ayurveda* that traditional healers knew intimately!

For a start, let us look at what *Prana* is as per the healing texts of India. *Prana* itself is described as the combination of the three biological humours of *agni* (fire, *pitta*), *soma* (water, *kapha*), *vayu* (wind, *vata*) as well as the three mental traits of *sattvas* (purity), *rajas* (agitation) and *tamas* (ignorance), the five senses and the soul - *Sushruta Samhita, Sharirasthana*, IV.3. Thus, true '*pranic healing*' involves (physical) methods of which pacify and heal these [note the final note relative to surgery].

The modern healer by contrast is an emotionalist that has 'picked up' such methods from a dubious Indian 'Guru' (usually influenced by western trends and superficiality and knowing little of real Yoga or Ayurveda outside these), at a weekend retreat, two week course etc. and feel they have picked up the powers to heal, apart from having no knowledge of Vedic sciences as Yoga, Ayurveda and others, of true healing therapies, herbs, diagnosis, treatment, examination etc. and also forget that such powers, even for the advanced spiritual aspirant within Vedic and Chinese traditions was itself a rarity over a common occurrence!

It is merely the western egotism that feels that it can pick up such modalities and powers that took decades and lifetimes of traditionalists to gain and simply validate themselves as if they are avatars born with such, but again unlike true avatars, are unable and unwilling to prove and substantiate their claims (apart from my attacking their questioning opposition bu shouting them down, again in Pentecostal manner like barking dogs!).

Sadly however, since the majority of Hindus since the 10th Century listened to the naive uneducated masses of merchants (*vaishyas*) and others who became teachers and Gurus and developed their own naive and blind faith-based traditions over Brahmanical logic and rationalism or sciences (i.e outside the sphere of traditional teachings, commentaries and integral sciences as atomism, cosmology, astronomy, mathematics and schools of debate, logic and reason), the scores of Indians have today embraced such nonsense when re-imported back into their own culture and are often unwilling to give these 'foreign' trends up and ironically, embrace them as tradition, ignoring history and their own classical references that speak otherwise (much how Indian Law and Hindu dogmatism today is based upon the draconian Victorian British system that has been replaced in Britain and other colonies); they ignore their own traditions and traditional authorities and instead, by "*conservative and traditional*", the modernist Hindu often refers to the prudish Victorian psyche or the reimported Americanised and New-Age traditions that has come to shape what to them is "tradition"!

Other trends such as *Chakra-Balancing* can be seen in the same light; as reconstituted and re-imported versions of indigenous Indian ideals that then become the mainstream in India. Such insidious traditions remind one of the "Dark Ages" in Europe that stiffed logic, reason, rationalism and science in Europe due to the power of the Church and its threats!

The *chakras* themselves on a physical level refer to no more than the geographic regions of the body that correspond to physical organs that are to be treated in a physical manner (via herbs, dietary regimes, detoxification by way of Ayurvedic clinical methods, herbal formulas or even surgical); internally they refer to the inner worlds or *lokas*, realms and spheres of consciousness which are accessed only by the 'A-Grade' and highest-level rare *Yogi* with his mind. Thus, the idea of balancing the *chakras* and other such is nonsense in the Yoga sphere; such also refer to the *mahabhutas* or cosmic elements, which cannot be manipulated by external application of hands, gems etc. as eople may think! *Mantras* were themselves were a more mental or placebo-manner employed, hence the term *mantra* itself derives from *manas* (the mind) - we shall discuss the psycho-somatic approach further down.

The average person clings to these naive beliefs as they have not and are unwilling to study the classical texts and historical traditions and instead try and validate their diminutive learning and defend it, as an aggressive Christian preacher does their precious Biblical verses (according to them to justify their lifestyles personally), the difference being the New-Agers wish to defend their invalid and useless Certifications and what it has cost them - often being their only examples of "validation" of their lifetime! Thus, like dear life, they cling onto it like glue!

A true reading of the classical Vedic texts untainted by naive *Vaishnava* dualism, western Christian influences or New Age hyperbole and according to traditional commentaries and etymologies reveal them to be rational and methodical in approach.

Indeed, while many 'testify' to the benefits of Reiki, Pranic Healing and such, the classical *shastras* of India see such as having mere placebo effects and hence the effects are purely psycho-somatic and not actually a reality. Understanding the mind, *Charaka Samhita* (*Sutrasthana, XI.46, 54*) states many ritualistic or "spiritual" therapies and rituals in the Vedic era were merely to keep the mind freed of unwholesome objects for the mind and hence their employment in treatment (*mano-nigraha* - attempts to subdue the mind). *Charaka* thus states that opposite therapies (rituals and specific meditations) according to the disorders of the psyche.

Unlike the delusional (*mudha*) and distracted (*vikshepa*) nature of the modern minds in New-Age circles that are (a) ignorant of and (b) reject the ancient and vast traditions of Yogic and Ayurvedic psychology and their in-depth views upon the mind, the ancient traditions understood the mind and its delusions well, including the effects of placebos!

My question to all such people practising Ayurveda, Yoga, Reiki, Pranic or Faith / Energy Healing etc. is, **"Do you understand Yogic and Ayurvedic Psychology, the levels of the mind and have you studied these to know the difference?"**. The answer is always something along the likes of emotions, feelings and personal self-hypnotised views that might as well be '*As Jesus came and told me so*' or as '*The Holy Spirit advised me*'.

One of the very reasons I started writing when I was 15 years old onwards, was to educate people in the true and proper Yogic traditions I have studied through various works, traditional texts and my own lineage that included several Scientist-Yogis and advanced Yogis and to also reveal to the world their teachings in a more simplistic form and explain the traditional explanations and vastness of the Vedic teachings, not merely their pasteurised and superstitious forms! This also includes the psychology of Yoga of which I have studied for years.

Patanjali in his *Yoga Sutras* notes of the strength of the mind by the maxim "as one thinks - one becomes" on this note:

"By performing samyama (yogic concentration) on the power of elephants, one can eve attain such a strength." (3.25)

Thus, even in an unconscious state, one can, if the desire is strong enough, believe in something and thus *feel* as if one is gaining the desired effects. Even though a pseudo-science, hypnosis itself proves this, by the power of suggestion!

As is thus warned in the *shastras*, "*as one thinks - that one becomes*" according to the inherit nature of his actions (*Bhagavad Gita*, 17.3-6). The entire 17th Chapter of the *Gita* is also with respect to the *gunas* through *karmas* (actions) and their impact upon shaping our *samskaras* (karmic impressions) and *vasanas* (mental impressions).

Likewise, the great monist *Shankaracharya* in his *Vivekachudamani* (113) states that *avriti* or the veiling power of the mind linked to the vitiation of the mind or *tamas* (darkness and ignorance of the mental channels) causes a failure to recognise the truth. This same fault of the mind he links to the soul's reincarnation due to *vikshepashakti* or the power of projection.

While these may be damning to the minds of those who both practice and take up such non-traditional "healing arts" that even within native traditions are considered "pseudo-sciences" practiced by the lesser classes as in India (as with the *Romani* or Gypsy that came from India into Europe and gave their corrupted Vedic traditions, influencing New-Age hysteria and trends) or other cultures outside the more educated classes as the Brahmins or Priests and *Acharyas* and *Shastris* - the true teachers and academics who see such as superstitious and illogical and not to mention, are also byproducts of the modern (European) mind that seeks to create some kind of 'spiritual renaissance' by adopting these foreign native traditions, despite that for example, even in the earlier *Tretayuga* of the Hindus (traditionally said to be millions of years ago), a more spiritual age than now that surgery and physical methods of healing came to replace herbal and spiritual cures alone as they, even long ago, became invalid!

While various spiritual therapies were employed in ancient times, these did not include anything like so-called *pranic healing* nor Reiki, but of ritualistic disciplines etc. that were viewed in a more rational manner as explained in the healing texts of *Ayurveda*, which remains a complete medical system, not simply an irrational spiritual healing system as many Americans believe today!

Charaka (*Charaka Samhita, Sutrasthana*, XI.46, 54) states even of these so-called "spiritual" therapies however, that such were used simply employed and developed as psychological tools to keep the mind freed of unwholesome objects or thoughts (such as from performing further negative actions, further complicating the disease or treatment) and hence their usage was purely placebo-based alone (*mano-nigraha* - that which subdues or restrains the mind), which constitutes the employment of the threefold Ayurvedic approach to healing:

-**Sattvavajaya** (methods by which *sattvas* or purity is increased in the mind) or psychological therapies - of which the next compliments...

-**Daivavyapashraya**, the "illuminating therapies" or psycho-somatic / placebo therapies hence form an integral part of and are done along with the next or

- **Yuktivyapashraya**, that is, rational therapies as diet, herbs and formulas for the mind.

Thus, treatment of both physical and psychological disorders in the texts are said to be by way of purification (*shodhana*), palliative measures (*shamana*) and dietary regimes and regulation (*aharachara*) - *Sushruta Samhita, Sutrasthana,* I.26-27, thus more physical, rational and practical treatments including clinical methods such as *Panchakarma* for detoxification, even in ancient times that were considered to be more spiritual ages by the Hindus.

Modern people in America that defend the 'New Age' Ayurveda that is commonly marketed and branded as traditional and authenic however ignore the traditional views and texts or references and have thus developed their own anti-surgical, anti-physical and quasi-spiritual system of healing that traditional Ayurveda in its complexity actually criticises.

Likewise, on *Shalyatantra* (surgery), it is said to be the primal and most important branch of *Ayurveda* through which even in ancient times was used for organ-transplants (*Sushruta Samhita, Sutrasthana* I.16-18) of which the first teacher of *Ayurveda* (*adideva*), Dhanvantari reincarnated to teach to humanity (ibid, 21). It is also this very text that gave us our modern science of plastic surgery that the British discovered in India in the 18th Century in Mysore in Southern India!

This was as in such times even in the *Treta-Yuga* of yore, that subtle or spiritual methods and herbs alone were not enough to heal the body and it came from an ancient lineage of primal surgeons (*Ashwins*) from the lineage of human progenitors (*Prajapati*) from the Supreme (*Brahma*). From the original surgeons, it is said that *Indra* learnt it and from him the original *Dhanvantari* who later took incarnation as the *Dhanvantari* or *Kashi* or Varanasi (*Divodasa*) - much as *Sri Krishna* in the *Mahabharata* is said to be the reincarnation of *Rishi Narayana* of *Badrinath*.

This leaves the question of spiritual and subtle modalities of healing on lesser *yugas* or epochs as our own today, in question and also questions their very so-called 'ancient origin'!

References:

-Sushruta Samhita

-Charaka Samhita

-Yoga Sutras

-Bhagavad Gita

III. Dispelling the Marma Misconceptions: The Fallacy of *Siddha*

Background:

"Herbs were generated in ancient times, three yugas before the deities. Of these, the brown-hued, I tell their one hundred and seven locations"
-Rig Veda Samhita, 10.97.1, Yajurveda, XVII.49

There are more evidences of subtle sciences in the *Rig Veda* that several *vaidyas* have also ignored, as the mention of all 107 I stated in *Rig Veda* as *Marma* is evidenced by *Yaskacharya* who commented thus on the *Rig Vedic* verse re marmas:

"Saptashatam purushya marmanam teshvena dadhatiti va"
-Nirukta, Daivata Kanda, 9.28

The 700 appears to denote the *Siras* or veins that run through the marmas in Ayurveda that some southern systems have seen as more or less as 700 marmas giving this confusion. The commentary on the *Rig Vedic* verse (X.97.1) which lists the 107 *Marmas* which I originally hypothesised, but here *Yaska* presents a clear-cut case for this at any rate!

I had noted before that the verse denotes the 107 Marmas in the body and the term *babru* relates to the brown medicines as *tailas* or oils respective to each. It appears from historicity, that *Yaskacharya* also sees the same and substantiates my view / claim here. New Age Ayurveda views *Marmas* (vital spots) as energy centres for activation and healing through acupressure, acupuncture or stimulation and also healed by methods such as Reiki and Pranic healing by laying the hands on the patient.

Traditionally, **Marmas** are vulnerable and require *varma* (armour / protection). They formed a part of the science of *Dhanurveda* and even the *Rigveda* gives many examples of how they are to be protected. Just as we have modern "New-Age" authorities, so India is also flooded with dubious references such as *Puranic* systems that don't agree with *shruti* (revealed) texts such as the four *Vedas*. We shall explain the rejection of *Vedic* compared to so-called *Siddha* systems in later times (in short, 'Siddha' systems are nothing more than Vedic; *Rig Veda* being *shruti* and reliable in Hinduism and having such *Rishis* such as *Agastya* composing hymns there reveals the Tamil traditions formed later and are thus divergent systems from the originals. *Sushruta* and others continue the *shrauta / Vedic* traditions, hence *su-shruta* (heard well), which are traced back to the systems of the *Ashwins* from the *Vedas* themselves.

For a start, *Sushruta Samhita* (*Sharirasthana*, VI, 41-43) states *marmas* should not be damaged in any way, which also means no use of acupressure nor acupuncture on them traditionally, as these cause damage and aggravate the *doshas* (and organs they relate to), which includes cutting, hitting, fire even near them causes issues (*Sushruta Samhita, Sharirasthana*, IV 35 & 41).

In his chapter on *Siras* or veins and venesection, *Sushruta* also states that one should avoid all areas where there are *Marmas* for this procedure also. This again alludes to the prohibition of acupressure and acupuncture at the Marma sites and shows they are to be avoided and not touched, except for healing purposes (when wounded due to battle, accidents etc.).

Marmas were hence used in battle for the purposes of maiming others and causing various injuries to organs they relate to and should be healed alone, not pushed, prodded or manipulated, which although can produce short-term effects, long-term, would aggravate the *doshas* and cause injuries to organs, as per the *Samhitas*. They hence formed a part of the science of *Dhanurveda* or Indian Martial Arts, which was taken to China by Buddhist monks around the 5th Century AD, along with Ayurveda, the science to heal them when they were impaired to avoid damage to the vital organs they corresponded to.

The *Rig Veda* (VI.75.18) states that one places armour or protection (*varma*) overs his *marmas* (vital points), which also stresses of the ancient importance of them being protected and not harmed in battle, as *Sushruta* also states later. Vedic warriors hence placed *varma* or protection over these regions, which naturally their opponents would seek to strike. This ancient martial-arts and medical knowledge of *marmas* hence dates back as far as the *Rigveda*, despite many citing references in *Atharvaveda* for it.

Originally, *Marmas* had their respective oils, pastes and formulas for healing them, reducing swelling (*sophahara*), healing wounds and pains (*vrana-ropana, shulahara*) etc. (as stated in *Rig Veda*, X.97.1). Originally, *Marmabhyanga* or *Marma-*Massage included therapies where *Tailas* or oils were used in the reduction of accumulation of *doshas* at the site of the *Marmas*; coconut-based oils and soothing pastes where *Pitta* and bleeding were involved, drying herbs and pastes where *Kapha* was involved with swelling and application of heat-boluses etc. to reduce swelling as also *Tailas* or oils for *Vata* where there was dryness and cracking at *Marma* sites to counter this - which also involves processes such as *Shirodhara* for the head-*marmas* (region of *Pranavayu*), when *Vata* invaded the head *Marmas* and so on.

The commentator on the *Sushruta Samhita*, *Dalhana* himself states the definition of *Marma* is "*Marayanti iti marmani*", which means that a *Marma* is one which causes death (if damaged).

Now, as a "Vedic rationalist", I also don't simply dismiss such, but in my own Ayurvedic clinical experience, I have found hundreds of patients, sometimes 12 - 20 years after receiving *marma-chikitsa* (*marma* therapy) or acupuncture, or damage near *marmas* (or to them), that the corresponding organs and systems have become impaired. For eye disorders, especially cataracts for example, several have had acupuncture on the feet (the classics are quite clear about massaging the feet for health but avoiding injury to them and hence use of sandals etc. to protect them and hence the eyes).

Yogic Healing of *Marmas* was done via various *Pranayamas* (breathing techniques) that had specific effects to reduce the aggravation of *doshas* (biological humours) in the body, not by energy-methods of healing. Massage (*abhyanga*) was done on a superficial level of touch and very softly with oils such as *Murivenna Taila, Vranaropana Taila, Jathyadi Taila / Ghrita, Dhanwantara Taila, Mahanarayana Taila etc.* (if wounded), as well as pastes especially those such as *Marma Gudika* (used topically as a paste and taken internally). Pastes and oils are also used to heal them as gentle massages (not acupressure or acupuncture). This is the fine-line between "pressure" and "healing" (as with any wounds or injuries; moving a fractured limb once set is hardly going to help in the healing process!).

The Myth of Siddha and Vedic: The Sinhalese Buddhist Origin

With reference to the *Vedas* as authority, some groups in the south claim that the *Vedas* were derived from the older *Pranava-Veda* that included the southern *Agamas* and hence point for the origin of acupuncture and acupressure to be thus validated. For a start, if such were true, the *Agamas* and the *Vedas* derived from them would include references to the positive (healing) effects of such, which we shall examine, they do not! Secondly, *Agastya* , who many claim is the originator of non-Vedic *Siddha* traditions is also a famous Seer in the *Rig Veda* along with his brother, *Vasishtha*.

Saivism itself pervades the *Vedas*; the *Yajur Veda* is devoted to *Shiva*, while other things associated with *Shiva* and the Yogic traditions in India are the great death mantra (*Mahamrityunjaya*), which asks the great god to deliver us from mortality to immortality. This mantra appears as a mantra of the Sage *Vasishtha* (brother of *Agastya*) in the *Rig Veda* (VII.59.12).

It appears however, that the South preserved the older side of the Vedic culture through the Brighu and Agastya Seers, whereas the North took upon newer recessions, such as the Shukla Yajur Veda or White Yajur Veda, through Yajnavalkya.

Yajnavalkya himself, also author of famous texts as *Shatapatha Brahmana* and the *Brihadaranyaka Upanishad*, which have yogic and mystic siddha-like sciences everywhere, descends from the older *Taittiriya* Tradition of the *Aruni Rishis*. These *Aruna Rishis* themselves, as the name suggests, seem to have originated in the South for a start, around *Arunachala*.

We also note that famous *Shaivite* chants such as *Shri Rudram,* and Vedic Solar Yoga, lie in the older *Taittiriya Samhita* also, and show the later correlation of this area, with Shiva. *Arunachala* is also the region of *Siddhas* and *Nathas*, who are said to dwell there. Could these be the ancient *Aruna Rishis* to whom Vedic Seers as *Yajnavalkya* and others looked back to?

Certainly, it seems to fit with the entire tradition, and shows that the *Siddhas* and *Nathas* were merely later versions of the *Rishis* of ancient Vedic times. The Vedic *Maruts* appear as the later *Siddhas* of Tamil traditions and are likewise connected to *Agastya* and *Vasishtha* in the *Rig Veda* - which again asserts the unity of *Siddha* and *Vedic* traditions - thus calling into question the later acupuncture and acupressure *marma* aspects "ascribed" to *Agastya* etc. as being DERIVATIVES of the original Tamil-Vedic traditions, not the originals (that the *Vedic* reflects).

Once again, it further asserts that the Dravidian people are just older "Vedic stock" or the proto-Aryans, as opposed to non-Aryans! In fact, the southern *Iyer Brahmins* etc. derive from *Arya*. The *Aryas* of the North simply continued Vedic teachings with the SAME *Rishis* and again, if such *marma* practices were *Siddha*, would be found in the Vedic literature, rather than later invented traditions.

What is more, *Manu* (the first Aryan) in *Bhagavata Purana* (VIII.24.13) is stated to have been a King called *Satyavraya* from the *Dravida* province (Southern India) who sailed North to avoid the floods, and to whom the *Matysa* (fish) incarnation of *Vishnu* appeared to (even in *Shatapatha Brahmana*). Note that *Dravida* in Vedic texts also referred to Indo-Aryan speaking regions of *Maharashtra* and *Gujarat* and hence never implied a "race" or linguistic group of people!

Agastya and *Brighu* Rishis in the *Rig Veda*, are also portrayed as being put in a *kumbha* (pot) to escape floods, by their father *Varuna*, the god of waters. *Agastya* in Southern tales, also escapes this same southern flood!

Getting back to *Manu* and *Ila*, we find in the text B*rihadaranyaka Upanishad* (VI.4.28) *Ila* mentioned as '*Maitravaruni*' meaning 'daughter of *Mitra* (Sun) and *Varuna* (Waters)'- showing she is cognate to both *Satyavrata* and *Vaivasvata* and connects the two, and shows the first '*Aryans*' or Vedic people came from Southern Indian practices.

All this reveals that the acupuncture and acupressure styles of *marma-therapy* were unorthodox in both Tamil and Vedic traditions; we should note here also that *Nimbarkacharya* (3096BC), *Shankaracharya* (509BC) down to *Ramanuja*, *Madhavacharya* and *Vallabhacharya* as also *Sri Ramana Maharishi, Narayana Guru* etc. who along with *Agastya, Bhrigu, Vasishtha* and others were all from Southern-India originally, the region where the so-called *Siddha* traditions of non-Vedic practices arose - yet all taught Vedic sciences! This hence brings into question the non-Vedic *Siddha* origin of these people who espouse such nonsense. The great *Shankaracharya, Chandrasekharendra Saraswati* in his works also noted the similarity of Tamil to Vedic Sanskrit and a similar common origin.

My personal opinion, based on evidences, is that the acupressure and acupuncture side South comes from the *Thiyyas*, who influenced the Tamil and so-called (antagonistic) *Siddha* traditions, but are the lower castes who didn't have knowledge of the Ayurvedic Samhitas. Originally these people were the Sinhalese Buddhist monks who migrated to Kerala and Tamil Nadu from North Malabar into Coimbatore and mixed with the local people and became folk-physicians. In earlier times, they included earlier monks as *Bodhidharma* that were Buddhist monks in southern India and were naturally antagonistic towards Vedic teachings (being Buddhist) and were not allowed into the Vedic fold. The *Thiyyas* today are still the main families of these (unorthodox) or divergent practices of *marma-chikitsa*.

Here we see a change in systems. Their system of Ayurveda hence became argued as "*Siddha*" as (being Buddhists) they opposed the Vedas in some ways, due to their Buddhist background, and was is quite of a more recent date. As a result, they developed the acupressure and acupuncture schools of Ayurveda, which are NOT part of the traditional *Ashtavaidya* system of Kerala, set up by *Vagbhata's* descendants (some state after retiring from *Sindh* he came to live there). Later, the *Nairs* and *Thiyyas* intermingled and produced this weird hodgepodge form of so-called "Kerala Ayurveda" today. The influence also extended into *Maharashtra* at times from these people in Northern *Karnataka*. Note here that the British, during the Mysore Wars, discovered the *Sushruta Technique* of rhinoplasty and otoplasty of which is stilled used today , evidence of *Sushruta's* oldest system still being used in the region!

Secondly, the *Thiyya* people only gained wider acceptance as true *Vaidyas* or Ayurvedic practitioners after their social liberation from being lesser castes and outcastes (*dalits*) after *Narayana Guru* (1856-1928) came about. Likewise, other modern trends such as women wearing the upper-Sari covering the breasts, said to have been a part of 'conservative' Indian culture for thousands of years (like *marma* nonsense) is well-known for have come in more recently - even in the 1920s, it was common for women in *Kerala* to go bare-chested!

Thus, after this period when the *Thiyyas* gained acceptance and were allowed into Hindu temples in the south of India and society became more liberal, their *marma* teachings gained more acceptance and the various *Ayurvedic* schools merged along with Tamil Nationalism in the eastern state, based upon the original *Sinhalese Buddhists* who settled there about 1,500 years ago and were the original *dalits* or outcastes with their Vedic-derisive systems fused with local *Brahmanical (Iyer)* teachings they had come into contact with. Hence the origin of the divergent Vedic *marma* systems and their later validated by "modern" Ayurveda circles.

Going Back to the Original Texts:

Now, before I have the "Tamil Nationalist" police on my tail, let me state that my father's side of my family is originally from Chennai. So, I am not some North-Indian that is speaking against southern traditions, as I am of mixed heritage myself (I feel the distaste of Tamil Nationalists right now, wishing to bag me as an "evil North-Indian"!).

In a hymn to the weapons of war in the *Rig Veda*, the mention of the *marmas* or vital-spots ("pressure points") – VI.75.18 and asks King (god) *Soma* and the armor (*varma*) to protect us.

It shows that pressure point blows and such a science does indeed, date back to the Vedas as the tradition shows, through the *Brighu* family Seers, an ancient Seer family as old as the Rig Veda. It reveals here however that the *marmas* were points that when pushed, pierce or maimed, they cause harm, not cures and hence pastes etc. were used to heal them.

Traditionally, the *Brighu* family's member, *Parshurama* or Rama *Jamadagni* is accredited with founding the martial science of *Dhanurveda* in India, and is especially related to Kerala, and its origin who derive from the *Kerala* region which was also historically ruled by *Mahabali*, the demon-King mentioned in connection with the *Trivikrama* form of *Vishnu* in the *Rig Veda*. *Parshurama* is also lauded in India as an avatar (incarnation) of the god Vishnu.

Moreover, these references appear in the Sixth *Mandala* (sixth book) of the *Rig Veda*, which are ascribed to another family of Seers, the *Bharadvaja* family of Seers, a sub-family of the *Angirasa* family. Seer *Bharadvaja* himself is one of the famous teachers of Ayurveda, as in later times through the *Charaka* lineage of Seers.

Along with the *Brighu* Seers, the *Angirasas* are also the other prominent family in the ancient *Rig-Veda* text, and of *Vedic* India.

To reiterate these claims, the *marmas* or vital-points of Indra's enemy is also mentioned in *Rig Veda* (III.32.4; V.32.5) in relation to wounding the enemy with the *vajra* (thunderbolt) or a weapon. The killing of the ninety-nine *Vritras* (obstructions) is also mentioned (I.84.13), perhaps relating to 99 *marma* points used in the battle. At any rate, it all reveals that *shuchi-karma* or piercing and pushing *marmas* as far back as the *Rig Veda* in which the later *Ayurvedic* traditions derive, is contraindicated. It is also proven in this article that the 107 classical *marmas* are well-known and dispels the myth of modern expounders to try and denigrate the term ""*marma*" used.

Other Classical References and Traditions:

Frank Ross in his book on Ayurvedic Acupuncture argues that the acupuncture arises even in *Sushruta Samhita* - but this is in reference to *raktamoksha* at the sites of *marmas*, for removing pus, swelling etc., not as a therapeutic measure by itself, or acupuncture as such! *Sira vedha* (venesection) is quite different from *suchi karma* or so-called needling! As noted, these anti-Vedic "*Siddhas*" are not even Tamil, but of Sinhalese Buddhist descent that came into the South around 200-300BCE and mixed with the locals and stole ideas such as Agastya etc. as their founder. Silly people today think its part of Tamil tradition, which is not, as that is the Brahmins of which *Agastya*, *Pulastya*, Vasishta have always been part of!

The fact remains that *marmas* are "vital points" are under no circumstances are me be damaged in any way, shape or form, but merely healed.

On this, Ayurvedacharya *Sushruta* himself notes (*Sharirasthana*, IV.42) that any injuries to *marmas* - mildly dangerous or not, causes injuries resulting in death or deformities of the body.

Now, relative to the "subtle" healing methods of *Marmas*, let us also note more following references from the *shastras* rather than divergent traditions of the hearsay of latter-day schools or "Vedic -derivatives".

Charaka (*Charaka Samhita*, *Sutrasthana*, XI.46, 54) states even of so-called "spiritual" therapies however, that such were used simply employed and developed as psychological tools to keep the mind freed of unwholesome objects or thoughts (such as from performing further negative actions, further complicating the disease or treatment) and hence their usage was purely placebo-based alone (*mano-nigraha* - that which subdues or restrains the mind), which constitutes the employment of the threefold Ayurvedic approach to healing:

-**Sattvavajaya** (methods by which *sattvas* or purity is increased in the mind) or psychological therapies - of which the next compliments...

-**Daivavyapashraya**, the "illuminating therapies" or psycho-somatic / placebo therapies hence form an integral part of and are done along with the next or

- *Yuktivyapashraya*, that is, rational therapies as diet, herbs and formulas for the mind.

Thus, treatment of both physical and psychological disorders in the texts are said to be by way of purification (*shodhana*), palliative measures (*shamana*) and dietary regimes and regulation (*aharachara*) - *Sushruta Samhita, Sutrasthana,* I.26-27, thus more physical, rational and practical treatments including clinical methods such as *Panchakarma* for detoxification, even in ancient times were considered to be more spiritual ages by the Hindus. This here, as with his other references (remembering, going back to the *Ashwini Ayurveda* systems of the *Rig-Veda / shrauta* traditions) would also call into question the *marma-healing* techniques of acupressure, acupuncture and pranic-healing of these sites as opposed to physical pastes, oils etc.

Modern people in America that defend the 'New Age' Ayurveda that is commonly marketed and branded as traditional and authentic however ignore the traditional views and texts or references and have thus developed their own anti-surgical, anti-physical and quasi-spiritual system of healing that traditional Ayurveda in its complexity actually criticises. Likewise, Tamil Nationalism in the South which has adopted an anti-Vedic psyche thanks to the British, also fails to address such, trying, like the New-Age sphere to reinvent its own "Siddha school" of Ayurveda, which is essentially no different to mainstream Ayurveda such as *Vagbhata's* system South (*Ashtavaidya*) in later times, just as great *Acharyas* as *Shankaracharya* and others were also from traditional southern regions!

Likewise, on *Shalyatantra* (surgery), it is said to be the primal and most important branch of *Ayurveda* through which even in ancient times was used for organ-transplants (*Sushruta Samhita, Sutrasthana* I.16-18) of which the first teacher of *Ayurveda* (*adideva*), *Dhanvantari* reincarnated to teach to humanity (ibid, 21). It is also this very text that gave us our modern science of plastic surgery that the British discovered in India in the 18th Century in Mysore in Southern India!

This was as in such times even in the *Treta-Yuga* of yore, that subtle or spiritual methods and herbs alone were not enough to heal the body and it came from an ancient lineage of primal surgeons (*Ashwins*) from the lineage of human progenitors (*Prajapati*) from the Supreme (*Brahma*). From the original surgeons, it is said that *Indra* learnt it and from him the original *Dhanvantari* who later took incarnation as the *Dhanvantari* or *Kashi* or Varanasi (*Divodasa*) - much as *Sri Krishna* in the *Mahabharata* is said to be the reincarnation of *Rishi Narayana* of *Badrinath*.

Remember here that *Indra* himself dates back to the oldest teachings of the so-called *Siddha* masters who were Vedic *Rishis*, wherein *Indra* uses piercing of marmas and such techniques to HARM his enemies, not heal them! Thus it is a continuous tradition, revealing all others are merely non-Vedic, non-traditional divergents, just as the Romani (Gyspies) are divergent versions of true Vedic-Hindu teachers or as various astrologers in India follow divergent non-original invented schools (if you like, the "ancient New-Age" techniques that had no historical basis nor validation in ANY scholarly or accepted traditions in India itself).

Hence, relative to arguments on *marmas*, we need to look deeper than merely the superficiality relative to healing, of which the tradition of the *Rig Veda* down to *Sushruta* etc. and commentators such as *dalhana* all agree that *marmas* are for protection, not pressing and prodding. Other views are thus *ashrauta* or not revealed and unorthodox; as noted, the texts themselves cite the importance of surgery, but also of keeping away from *marmas* during such invasive practices also!

References:

- Durgadas (Rodney) Lingham, **Arya Nyaya Rahasya**: Academy of Traditional Ayurveda, 2015

- Sushruta Samhita

- Charaka Samhita

- Nirukta

- Rig Veda Samhita

IV. Meats and their Use in Ayurveda

Many are also unaware that great Swamis such as Swami Vivekananda also ate meat, including beef! Sri Aurobindo also ate fish and chicken in his earlier days - both Vivekananda and Aurobindo were Bengalis, where the main staple is fish. Yet, many ignore this as also with others historically in addition to classical health reasons in the texts that sometimes require meat, whereas the modern New-Age Ayurveda paradigm rejects such and long-term, ignores medical concerns from both a western and Ayurvedic perspective and insteda superimposes its own limited understanding and biases in an attempt to ignore and even thwart traditional views.

The reason I began writing on such is due to the common misconceptions we see in the western world. As a traditionally trained practitioner, I had teachers ranging from BAMS graduates to those who had spent several decades in family traditions. Both however had a strong zeal for classical references and influences as also tradition, which along with my own Vedic family background that sought to 'go back to the sources' (classics and native traditions), culminated in my questioning many aspects of what has come to epitomise Ayurveda in the western world today.

Most diseases in Ayurveda are of *Vata* (gas-increasing and dry) origin which are aggravated by raw foods, especially beans, leafy greens etc. Vegetables need to be spiced and cooked in oils like ghee or sesame to reduce them. This IS NOT just a constitutional issue - old age, cold climates, A/C offices and even our fast-paced lifestyles aggravate *Vata* in almost everyone! Such raw-food and high-dairy and heavy diets are suitable for those with a higher bilious constitution or *rajasic* or passionate-nature, such as active people (warriors, dancers etc.) such as we see in ancient India with the diets of **Hatha-Yoga**, that also included many practices such as the *shat-shuddhi-kriyas* (six actions of purification) that could in normal people, cause disturbances due to their non-therapeutic and harsh actions on the body. The classics also warn of this as well. Such are different to the tailored approach of systems such as *Panachakarma*in Ayurveda and cannot be taken in the same light for healing.

Yoga traditionally required many abdominal and other exercises and regimes (as *basti* or enemas) that helped increase one's bodily *jatharagni* (digestive fire) and other *dhatvagnis* (metabolism of the tissues) which helped absorb the more *sattvic* or pure foods they consumed, which were aimed at purity of the mind for meditation techniques and spiritual life, such as avoiding passion-increasing foods to withholding their *ojas* or bodily vitality through *brahmacharya* or celibacy. For the average person, such as Ayurveda addresses, the case was different - and hence the sciences such as *vajikarana* or aphrodisiacs was an important one, that itself often used animal products and formulas in its formulas for people in the mainstream of society for better health and vitality, outside the monastic Yogi communities. Still, there were also householder Yogis, of which many of the *Ayurvedic Rishis* or Seers themselves derived!

We should note that *Krishnamacharya*, the brother-in-law of *BKS Iyengar* was an *Ayurvedic Vaidya* or Practitioner and gave out specific, not generic regimes relative to Yoga after a full Ayurvedic examination of the person, dietary regimes etc. He himself had trained with one of the original people Hatha-Yoga itself created - the *Gurkhas* of Nepal!

The classics give numerous elaborate descriptions as per the properties of various meats - especially for their Vata-reducing properties. Those such as peacock for example were commonly used for improving eyes, voice, intellectual capabilities, complexion, hearing etc. and was commonly used. Goat-meat was also well-known for bulking the tissues and often used as a meat-soup or even *basti*(enema). Goat and mutton are said to be strengthening or tonifying for the body, and so good for Vata people and severe debilitated conditions (*Ashtanga Hridayam, Sutrasthana,* VI.63-64). Goat also does not cause malas or wastes in the body (*Charaka Samhita, Sutrasthana,* XXVII.61).

Likewise, beef is said to cure dry cough, exhaustion, chronic nasal catarrh, emaciation and excess hunger (*Ashtanga Hridayam, Sutrasthana,* VI.65).

Swans, iguana, sparrow, quail, hare, buffalo, tortoise, rhinoceros and others are discussed by *Charaka* and others, while some texts discuss the properties of exotic meats such as tigers, lions, frogs, porcupines and others (that are mentioned in classics as *Charaka* but not elaborated upon).

The ancient author *Sushruta* in the *Sushruta Samhita* (*Sutrasthana,* XLVI.351-365) also mentions the various ways in which meats can be cooked and taken and their own therapeutic actions as a result of these, including soups, minced-meat, roasted and those cooked with herbs etc. and their specific actions accordingly.

Charaka Samhita (Sutrasthana, XXVII) notes the various therapeutic qualities of meats:

Goat doesn't vitiate the *srotas* or bodily channels and is *brimhana* (tonifying), as also is mutton.(61-62)

Peacock meat is good for eye-sight, hearing faculties, promotes intellectual abilities, improves the digestive fire, good for age (aging disorders), complexion, voice and also for promoting life-force (*ayu*) as well as helping improve reproductive fluid in males and is tonifying. (64-65)

Chicken is warming in nature, tonifying to the body, provides virility, is tonifying to the body (bulking), awakens the voice, provides strength and greatly reduces *vata* in the body as well as causes sweating. (66-67)

Pork is fleshy, strengthening to the body, creates brightness of the skin, is oily and heavy, tonifying, grants virility and vitality to the body, alleviates exhaustion (chronic fatigue) and reduces and pacifies *vata*. (78-79)

Beef is useful in disorders where there is complete *vata*, rhinitis, intermittent fevers, cough, wasting disorders, vitiation of muscle mass and for excess digestive fire (in cases of over-eating etc.). (79-80)

Fish are oily, warming in nature, sweet in taste and help strengthen and tonify the body as well as alleviate *vata*. (81-82)

Eggs of peacocks, chickens and swans are said to be useful in vitiation of semen, coughs, heart disorders as well as in accidental injuries and don't cause too much heat in the body, are sweet in taste and provide strength to the body. (86-87)

It should also be noted that people in southern India in the state of Kerala, including Hindus commonly eat beef. While there are strict Brahmins who don't engage in any meats and not even onions and garlic (being considered *rajasic* foods), nonetheless, this practice is widespread. The Vedic text *Shatapatha Brahmana* (III.1.2.21) notes of the sanctity of beef, but the author, *Rishi Yajnavalkya* states that he eats beef if the meat is considered tender. *Brihadaranyaka Upanishad* (VI.4.18) similarly states that if one desires a strong offspring that can recite the Vedas properly a dish of boiled rice, ghee and meat should be taken by husband and wife, preferably beef or veal.

In the Vedic period, people were spiritual and also rational. Meat-eating was not abused, but animals were sacrificed at times according to various purposes and desires, such as *rajasic* (passionate) ones, by both Brahmins and *kshatriyas* alike. Meats were taken in sacrifice to avoid karma of killing the animals and ensuring a better future life for them. Others in more *sattvic* or pure modes however would partake only in meat-substitutes in the form of *rasayanas* or rejuvenation formulas. Much here appears to be dependent on *gotras* or seer families; for health purposes, it appears quite clear that partaking in meat outweighed the need for keeping animals alive (over humans).

What is *tamasic* for one is *sattvic* for others. The Yogic diets have been long-created and established in various lineages and those outside required more *pitta* constitutions to get used to these; other types would fail, which is why more *rajasic* and *pitta* types took up *Hatha-Yoga* and such diets. *Vata* types for example suffer from hyperactivity and oscillate between hyper and hypo-metabolic functions and need warming and heavier foods, such as meats provide to slow them down (make them (*tamasic* or stop their excesses), whereas *pitta* types already have a sharp fire, are very *rajasic* and active in metabolic and mental faculties and require more *sattvas* and hence *sattvic* foods work best for them; *kapha* types fall in between and lack energy and dynamism and suffer from hypometabolic conditions and hence need more stimulating or *rajasic* foods such as spices and such to get their digestions, minds and bodies going and warm their dense and cold natures up!

Thus, *sattvic* foods for each type actually differs greatly and the rigid Yogic (stereotypical *sattvic*) diet fails when liberally applied to one and all. Some require meats and others do not. *Vata* types are most likely to require meats, while the other two types do not.

Charaka Samhita (*Sutrasthana*, XXVII, 311) states that good quality meats are *brimhana* (strengthening and building) as also *balya* (promoting strength). It states of meat-soups (*mamsarasa*) as one of the best for the body - that they are *sarvarogaprashamanam* (alleviates all diseases) and promotes *vidya*(wisdom), *swarya* (good voice), strength (*bala*) of *vayas* (age), *buddhi* (intellect), *indriyas* (senses) respectively (ibid, 314).

The texts therefore do not get carried away with meats and note cases where the excesses of meats are also noted. *Charaka* (*Chikitsasthana*, IX.96) also states that insanity can be avoided if one abstains from eating meats and wines or impure diets etc. and hence these substances are seen as causative factors (*nidanas*) of various kinds of insanity. Various meats and alcohol are given various factors or qualities (*gunas*) in Ayurveda, according to their chemical reactions upon the mind, which are described as aggravating *rajas* and *tamas* in the mental channels, blurring our perceptions. As such, they are to be avoided in such conditions where mental disorders are present. Muscular tumours and cancers result due to excess eating of meats (*Ashtanga Hridayam, Uttarasthana, 29; Bhava Prakasha, Madhya Khanda, III.44.22-23, Madhava Nidana, XXXVIII.22-23*).

As noted, relative to the mind however, while meats are avoided for meditation and psychological issues, in some cases where there is hyperactivity (a *vata* predominance), sometimes *guru* (heavier), snigdha (uctuous) and *ushna* (heating) substances are required to help "ground" *vata* (which is composed of subtle elements as air and ether). Many meats on this note are classified as having a *kapha* (water and earth) or increasing and bulking qualtity that helps ground the subtle elements of ether and air (*vata*) - having a more *parthiva* (earthly) element, giving stability to their fragile and light-weight bodies, thereby calming their overactive minds and imaginations. For disorders of the mind in more *pitta*(fire and water) and *kapha* (water and earth) types however, meats can aggravate their conditions by their unctuous, heating and heavier natures and thus best avoided for them (though again such depends on predominating elements in people and their *vikara* or vitiation on a case by case basis, not a generic model).

Historically, beef in India was consumed from bulls, the cow being seen as more useful for giving milk, from which ghee (clarified butter), curd, butter, cream etc. could be used

by ancient Hindus. Heavier meats are also heavier for digestion (horse, pork, beef etc.) in Ayurveda, which can also be seen to give rise to diseases due
to accumulation of *ama* or toxins, as we have noted above - and thus also more likely to cause psychological issues to to their difficult metabolism. Fish, lamb, goat, chicken and other birds were hence the 'main staple' of people in India as a result and beef was thus rarely consumed - the same for pork etc. which were heavier.

This also ties in with another historical reason why Indians ate less meat - diabetes. Today, India is the 'diabetes capital of the world'[3]. Historically also, Type 2 diabetes was a major issue in India owing to the high concentration of sweets and dairy consumed in India - remembering that ancient Indians preferred a lacto-vegetarian diet and high concentration of dairy within that, as also the originator of sugar for the world through the Roman trade-links from ancient times. The 'sweet tooth' of India is also why Type 1 and Type 2 diabetes are first described in Ayurvedic texts and as such, heavier foods such as meats would only complicate matters and increase *kapha* (phlematic humour), already increased in India due to the excessive dairy and sweet foods historically consumed.

In saying this, again, there are numerous diseases in Ayurveda where meats are used. There are also various Hindus in India that eat meats as well, such as the *Bengalis* in the East of India - it is also well-known that *Bengali Brahmins* also consume eggs; in regions to the east as in Assam, the sacrifice of goats, as also in Bengal to the Goddess has been an ancient custom and hence consumption of goat-meat, as is also common in the Himalayan region such as the consumption of goat and lamb by *Kashmiri Pandits*.

The traditional Ayurvedic model of the use of meats may hence be shocking to many in the west educated under American Ayurveda regimes, but is not to those traditionally trained in India or BAMS graduates who understand these therapeutic uses of meats and their application. There are many classical formulas and preparations that would also shock the average American Ayurvedic practitioner whose methods have come to represent a quasi-Buddhist system of vegetarianism over the original model.

This sadly also does not do justice relative to true healing as per Ayurveda, any more than the rejection of surgery in the modern (pseudo New-Age) American Ayurveda model employs - itself not even accessing the basic levels of true *Panchakarma* (five actions of *shodhana* or purification) which emphasises
not *Panchakarma* or *shodhana* but merely *shamana* or traditional palliative therapies in their pasteurised form (or Spa Ayurveda), which causes many misinterpretations about such systems and specifics - many of these even pasteurised and hemogenised versions of *purvakarma*(preliminary therapies) - again with generic substances used over specifics in tradition and diseases also classified into

[3] http://timesofindia.indiatimes.com/life-style/health-fitness/health-news/India-is-the-diabetes-capital-of-the-world/articleshow/50753461.cms//

simplistic *vata, pitta* and *kapha* categories and treated with generic decoctions and formulas.

References:

Durgadas (Rodney) Lingham: ***Aushadh Rahasya: The Secret of Ayurvedic Herbs and Disorders of the Mind: Lulu Publications, 2013***

- *Charaka Samhita*

- *Sushruta Samhita*

- *Ashtanga Hridayam*

- *Madhava Nidana*

- *Bhava Prakasha*

- *Sarngadhara Samhita*

GLOSSARY:

Agni – Fire. Also a Vedic God

Agni-Hotra – Vedic fire sacrifice or ritual

Aham - The Divine "I am", meaning "I am the Self". Synonymous with So'Ham.

Ahamkara - Ego. It is "I-ness" or the "I am the body" ideal.

Aksharas – The letters of the Sanskrit alphabet

Asana – A seat. Refers to Yogic postures.

Asura - Anti-God or dark force. In the older Vedic texts, a Mighty or Supreme God of Cosmic Power.

Atman - Self or Self

Atmajnana - Self knowledge / Wisdom of the Self

Atmavidya - Self wisdom

Avidya - Ignorance

Ayurveda - The 'Science of Life'. India's ancient medical tradition.

Bhakti – Devotion. Refers to the Yoga of Devotion.

Bhava – State (of consciousness), or attitude / temperament.

Bhutagnis – The fires of the *Bhutas* or *Panchamahabhutas* in Ayurveda

Bhutas – Also known as *Panchamahabhutas*, the five great elements of nature, *viz.* *akasha* (ether), *vayu* (wind), *agni* or *tejas* (fire), *jala* or *apas* (water) and *prithivi* (earth or gross matter).

Brahma - The Creator-God. One of the Hindu Trinity of Brahma, Vishnu and Shiva. He represents rajas (passion).

Brahman - The Supreme / Absolute Reality

Buddhi - The Intellect, source of mental digestion or metabolism.

Chitta - General term for the Mind. Specifically, it is the "Mind-stuff" or Unconscious mind.

Deva - Deity or Divinity, a God.

Devi - The Goddess

Dhatu – Bodily tissue; there are seven in Ayurveda. viz. *rasa* (plasma), *rakta* (blood), *mamsa* (muscle), *medas* (adipose), *majja* (nerves), *ashthi* (bone) and *shukra* (reproductive tissue).

Dhatvagnis – The seven fires of the bodily tissues

Dharana – Yogic concentration

Dhyana – Yogic meditation or contenplation

Dvaita - Dualism, doctrine of Dualism in Vedanta.

Dosha - Biological Humour - one of Vata (Wind), Pitta (Bile) or Kapha (Phlegm)

Graha – An Planet.

Granthi – Knot in Yoga. Also means a tumour.

Guna - Mode of Nature: sattvas, rajas and tamas and also the twenty attributes in nature also.

Hari - Vishnu, the preserver-god

Hatha Yoga – The Forceful Yoga of medieval India

Hridaya - Heart

Indra - Vedic God of the Self and Yoga, like later Shiva. Also represents *Vata dosha*

Japa – The chanting of mantras

Jatharagni – The digestive fire or metabolism

Jiva / Jivatman - Individual Soul or Self. Refers to the state where one has not yet realised the Soul's oneness with the Supreme.

Jnana - Wisdom or Knowledge. Also refers to Jnana Yoga, the path of Knowledge.

Jyotisha – Hindu Astrology

Karana (Sharira) - *also called* Linga Sharira. Causal body

Karma - Work or action. It is of three types - Sanchita, Accumulated; Prarabdha - that manifesting and Agami - Being created.

Kapha - Phlegm. The Water-humour in Ayurveda

Kosha – Bodily sheath. These number five – *Annamayakosha* (food sheath), *Pranamayakosha* (breath sheath), *Manomayakosha* (mental sheath), *Vijnanamayakosha* (wisdom sheath) and *Anandamayakosha* (bliss sheath)

Kriya - Works, Practices (especially in relation to Yoga)

Manas - The Mind. Specifically, the emotional mind.

Mandagni – The sage of the low / dull (*manda*) digestive fire.

Maya - Creation as the material world, seen as an Illusion and power of the great Goddess. It is like dream-substance.

Nadi – Relates to the pulse in Ayurveda and also the meridians in the body as well. It also means a river

Nadi-Pariksha / Nadi Vijnana - Pulse diagnosis or examination and wisdom in Ayurveda

Niyama – The yogic codes of conduct or right living

Ojas – Vitality or strength referring to the immune system and vigour in Ayurveda

Panchamahabhutas - Or Bhutas. Five Elements - Gross forms of Tanmatras: *Akasha* (Ether); *Vayu* (Wind); *Agni* (Fire); *Jala* (Water), *Prithivi* (Earth)

Para - Highest or Transcendental

Parakarana – Transcendental body

Paramatma - Supreme Self or Brahman. The state also of the Self in the Supreme Brahman.

Parambrahman – The Supreme Brahman or Great Being.

Pitta - Bile, the Fire-humour in Ayurveda

Pooja – Ritualistic offering or worship of the Gods.

Prarabdha - The Karma that exists due to previous samskaras or tendancies and comes out in the present body.

Prakriti - Nature. In Ayurveda, it means one's own Nature or Biological Constitution. It is also the Primal Nature from which creation itself is manifested through Maya.

Prana – Breath, Life-force. Also the Self. In Ayurveda, the form of Vata in the head-region

Pranayama – Breath control. Yogic breathing

Pratyahara – Withdrawing of the senses or control of impressions in Yoga

Purusha – The Cosmic Man or the Supreme Self. Cognate with Brahman.

Rajas / Rajasic - Quality of Passion, Ego, Pride, Desire, Movement and Agitation in Yoga. One of the Three Gunas or Modes of Nature.

Rishi - Ancient Seer or Wise Man.

Samagni – Stage of the equalised and good digestive fire

Samadhi – Yogic trance or absorption

Samkhya - The Hindu system of enumeration or cosmology

Samskara - Karmic residue or impressions

Sattvas / Sattvic - One of the Three Gunas or modes of nature in Yoga. Represents Truth, Purity, Clarity and Goodness.

Shankaracharya - Famous reformer of Hinduism and proponent of non-dualistic (Advaita) Vedanta, c.500bce. It was due to him that the Gupta Kings at the time of the Greeks practised Hinduism not Buddhism.

Shakti - Wife of Shiva and Goddess of Power. It is also Atma-shakti, the power of the Self, from which the world of manifestation of Maya comes from by reflection of it's energy or power

Sharira – Body. *See also* Sthula, Sukshma, Karana

Shiva - Yogi God of India responsible for Universal dissolution. One of the Hindu Trinity of Brahma, Vishnu and Shiva, representing tamas or inertia.

Smarana - Memory

Sthula (Sharira)– Physical or Gross body

Soma – The Vedic God representing *Ojas* or vitality and also the Moon

Sukshma (Sharira)– Subtle body

Tamas / Tamasic - One of the Three Gunas or modes of nature in Yoga. Represents the quality of Darkness, Inertia, Destruction and Ignorance.

Tanmatras - Subtle forces of the elements: Sound (Shabda), Touch (Sparsha), Sight (Rupa) , Taste (Rasa), Smell (Gandha)

Tiksagni – Form of Agni as the "sharp-penetrating" digestive fire.

Vasana - Mental Impression

Viveka – Discrimination. Also *Vivekagni*, the Fire of discrimination.

Vedas - "Wisdoms", ancient texts of India: Rig (Hymns), Sama (Songs), Yajur (Ritualism), Atharva (Occultism).

Vedanta – Hindu metaphysics

Vata - Wind, the Wind-humour in Ayurveda. Also means Wind.

Vayu - Wind or Air. Synonymous with Vata in Ayurveda.

Vishamagni – Stage of the variable or inconsistent digestive fire

Viveka - Discrimination

Vedanta - The philosophical system of India. Advaita (non-dualism) and Dvaita (dualism) are two opposites.

Yamas and Niyamas – Yogic restraints and codes of conduct

Yantra – Geometrical designs as a sacred image used for the deities along with mantras in their worship

Yoga - "Union", the system of Yoga

Yajna - Sacrifice, usually a Fire sacrifice (Hawana / Homa).

Bibliography:

Dr. David Frawley, *Ayurveda and the Mind: The Healing of Consciousness*: Lotus Press, Twin Lakes, Wisconsin, 2007

Dr. David Frawley, *Yoga and Ayurveda: Self Healing and Self-Realisation*: Lotus Press, Twin Lakes, Wisconsin, 2009

Swami Madhavananda, *Sri Shankaracharya's Vivekachudamani*: Advaita Ashram, India, 2009

Swami Muktibodhananda: *Hatha Yoga Pradpika*

Ram Kumar Rai, *Kularnava Tantra*: Prachya Prakashan, Varanasi - 221007, India, 1999

Prof. K.R. Srikantha Murthy, *Madhava Nidana:* Chowkhamba Krishnadas Academy, Varanasi, 2007

Prof. K.R. Srikantha Murthy, *Bhavaprakasha of Bhavamishra (Two Volumes)*: Chowkhamba, Krishnadas Academy, Varanasi, 2004

Prof. K.R Srikantha Murthy, *Sarngadhara Samhita*: Chowkhamba Krishnadas Academy, Varanasi,2007

Prof. K.R Srikantha Murthy, *Sushruta Samhita*: Chowkhamba Krishnadas Academy, Varanasi, 2007

Prof. K.R. Srikantha Murthy, *Vagbhata's Ashtanga Hridayam (Three Volumes)*: Chowkhamba, Krishnadas Academy, Varanasi, 2009

P.V. Sharma, *Charaka Samhita (Four Volumes*); Chowkambha Orientalia, Varanasi, 2011

Classical Texts:

Valmiki Ramayana

Hatha Yoga Pradipika of Swami Swatmarama

Vivekachudamani of Shankaracharya

Patanjali Yoga Sutras

Sushruta Samhita

Charaka Samhita

Ashtanga Hridayam

Madhava Nidana

Sarngadhara Samhita

Bhava Prakasha

Samkhya Karika of Ishvara Krishna

Nirukta and Nighantu

Vaisheshika Sutras

Madanpala's Nighantu

Hatha Yoga Pradipika

Rig Veda Samhita

Nirukta of Yaskacharya

www.ingramcontent.com/pod-product-compliance
Lightning Source LLC
Chambersburg PA
CBHW062342280526
45787CB00012B/586